The Unstoppable
Fat Loss Formula

DISCLAIMER

The ideas, concepts and opinions expressed in this book are intended to be used for educational purposes only. This book is sold with the understanding that the author and publisher are not rendering medical advice of any kind, nor is this book intended to replace medical advice, nor to diagnose, prescribe or treat any disease, condition, illness, or injury. It is imperative that before beginning any diet, nutrition, or exercise program, including any aspect of The Unstoppable Fat Loss Formula program, you receive full medical clearance from a licensed physician.

Author and publisher claim no responsibility to any person or entity for any liability, loss, or damage caused or alleged to be caused directly or indirectly as a result of the use, application, or interpretation of the material in this book.

Yes, the legal geeks made us print that!

The Unstoppable Fat Loss Formula

For information about Fit Body Boot Camp or to find one close to you see below:

Edited by Elaine Maxell

Top Fitness Articles, Inc.

Created by Bedros Keuilian and Fit Body Boot Camp

Designed and arranged by Adam R. Ake

Email: questions@fitbodybootcamp.com

Website: fitbodybootcamp.com

Phone number: (888) 638-FBBC (3222)

Address: 14788 Pipeline Avenue
Suite B
Chino Hills, CA 91709

To order additional copies of the Unstoppable Fat Loss Formula visit our website at: unstoppablefatlossformula.com

Meet Fit Body Boot Camp President

Bedros Keuilian

With over 15 years of experience in the fitness industry, Bedros Keuilian is the Founder and CEO of Fit Body Boot Camp, Inc., a global fitness boot camp franchise with locations in the U.S., Canada, the United Kingdom and Australia.

Bedros started out his career as a personal trainer. Along the way, he had the fortunate opportunity to successfully transition his experience into opening and operating a chain of personal training facilities in Southern California.

His success allowed him to parlay his experiences into helping other fitness professionals refine and grow their personal training businesses. Bedros recognized that personal trainers needed more effective marketing, sales and business systems. To service this need, Bedros developed multiple programs, resources and technologies which have helped thousands of fitness businesses market, grow and scale their personal training businesses.

Bedros has coached, taught, mentored, and supported over 6,500 fitness professionals worldwide helping many achieve six, multiple six and even seven figure generating businesses. He saw that the "next big thing" in the fitness industry would be the combination of personal training with boot camp workouts to create group personal training, which is the basis of *Fit Body Boot Camp's Unstoppable Fitness Formula* and its success in transforming lives worldwide, one client at a time.

A Word from Bedros

Why did I set out to write a book about fat loss? It's not like there's a vacuum when it comes to books on how to diet. But this is NOT another diet book!

I wrote this book to show *you* how to change your lifestyle; to teach you how to choose the correct foods that will turn your body into a fat burning machine. The strategy you'll find between these two covers is that of a complete lifestyle change– NOT a crash diet.

I'd like to personally welcome you to the Fit Body Boot Camp family.

At Fit Body Boot Camp our vision is…

As one of the fastest growing global brands in the group fitness and personal training industry, Fit Body Boot Camp's Global Goal by 2020 is to expose and engage 20% of the world's population to a healthy and fit lifestyle.

We can only accomplish this by continuing to innovate what we do, how we do it, and by being passionate about helping people achieve their fitness, fat loss, and health goals. We are laser-focused in mentoring successful Franchise Owners by helping them cultivate, develop, and foster long-lasting and loyal relationships with their end-clients by ensuring that they are passionate in who they are, what they do, and how they do it.

Fit Body Boot Camp's fun corporate culture and Core Values promote friends, family, and community and serve as the foundation for us to continue to deliver the "wow" factor that is global in reach, yet local in delivery. That is the Fit Body Boot Camp Way.

Fit Body Boot Camp Culture and Core Values:

Doing business should be fun. And it just makes sense that we treat our Franchise Owners and their clients like family. It's like the Golden Rule says; treat others like you want to be treated.

Our 10 Core Values that define us:

- Inspire fun and deliver happiness

- Be determined and driven

- Take pride in ownership

- Be nimble and decisive

- Instill confidence

- Be humble

- Embrace, encourage and drive change

- Cultivate a positive team and family culture

- Exceed the client's expectations

- Communicate openly and honestly

I applaud you on your quest for health and fitness and am confident that you'll meet your goals.

Please reach out to your local Fit Body Boot Camp location for support. We are your home for fitness and fat loss.

To your success,

Bedros Keuilian

Go online to
www.fitbodybootcamp.com/mealplans
to access:

Daily Caloric Intake Calculator
Alternative Vegetarian and Paleo Meal Plans
Grocery Lists

CHAPTER ONE

The Unstoppable Fat Loss Formula

What is the Unstoppable Fat Loss Formula?

- The Unstoppable Fat Loss Formula is a delicious way of eating that promotes healthy weight loss.

- It is a lifestyle to adapt, not a crash diet that causes you to revert back to your regular eating habits.

- And it is an active life with 3 to 5 boot camp workouts per week to keep motivation and metabolism high.

This is NOT a fad diet.

For more than 20 years the media has bombarded us with a perpetual diet craze. An avalanche of fad diets are announced one after another as breaking news while producing zero true results.

Sure, you may lose 5, 10, or even 20 pounds on a fad diet…but you'll gain it all back and then some. How can I be so confident that your results will be short lived? It's actually a simple concept and once you understand it you will be forever saved from the tortures of yo-yo dieting.

Fad diets saddle you with unreasonable calorie restrictions and some even cut out entire food groups just to produce that short lived drop in weight—a process that is actually harmful to your health. The fad diets also ignore one major component to shaping up: exercise.

You see, most fad diets operate on one age-old premise: **cut calories, cut calories, cut calories.** By restricting the type and amount of food consumed, the fad dieter usually sees an immediate drop in weight. If only it stopped there…

But it doesn't stop there. Life continues and the fad dieter returns to their pre-diet eating habits—with one major difference in their body due to the sudden drop in pounds. **Their calorie requirements have gotten smaller.**

In practical terms this means that the dieter will begin gaining weight even though they are eating their normal pre-diet portions. And since exercise hasn't become a part of their routine, the unneeded calories will result in pounds gained. So what's a dieter to do? Find a brand new diet to follow—right? Wrong.

There *is* a way to drop pounds and firm your body, but you won't read about it in the next diet book or hear it on the news. **The solution to your fad-dieting nightmare is a lifestyle change.**

What is a lifestyle change? To change your lifestyle means to replace unhealthy habits with healthy ones, and to do so consistently. It isn't something you do for a week or two, only to revert back your old ways—**a lifestyle change redefines who you are.**

I know this is starting to sound like some heavy stuff, but hear me out. Changing your lifestyle from one that is unhealthy to one that is healthy will be the best thing that you ever do for yourself. Trust me, I help people like you make this change every day with amazing results.

Your Lifestyle = Your Body

Fact: The shape of your body is the direct result of your current lifestyle.

So how do I change my lifestyle? That is a great question, and the answer is actually easier than you might think.

Most people who are unhappy with their bodies are really only holding on to a few bad habits. Once these destructive habits are identified and then replaced with healthy habits their body naturally transforms from one they loathe to one they are proud of.

In other words, to get the body you want simply determine your unhealthy habits and replace them with healthy ones. Here are the most prevalent unhealthy habits:

The habit of inactivity. Failing to exercise on a consistent basis is one of the most destructive obstacles for your health and figure. (The key word here is consistent. If you aren't exercising at least 3-4 times each week then you own this habit.)

The habit of overeating. Consuming calories in excess of your daily caloric needs is one of the main reasons that more adults are overweight today than ever before.

The habit of empty calories. Filling your diet with foods that hold little to no nutritional value is a great way to expand your waist. (Hint: if a food item is made up of mainly sugar and/or fat consider it 'empty' calories.)

You **can** lose weight and improve both your appearance and your health.

You **can** look and feel great.

You **can** transform yourself into the person that you've always wanted to be.

Don't let another day go by that leaves you a slave to unhealthy habits. Take action now.

By the way, I should mention another deadly habit that destroys too many people's dreams - **The habit of procrastination.**

How many times have you told yourself that you will start eating healthy tomorrow?

How many times have you promised that you would start an exercising program?

Each day that you succumb to the habit of procrastination is a day that pulls you farther and farther from your goals.

Break that nasty habit of procrastination—commit to *The Unstoppable Fat Loss Formula.*

What's Lifestyle Got To Do With It?

It happens to everyone.

That moment when you realize that it's time to do something about your weight.

It may happen when you're looking in the mirror, standing on the scale, or see a picture of yourself.

Your first thought is to go on a 'diet' but as quickly as that enters your mind the ghosts of a hundred diets past return…along with all the frustration.

Then you wonder, why bother?

The weight will come back, as it always has. Then you'll be back in front of the mirror discouraged as ever.

The answer is not to go on another diet.

The answer is to change your lifestyle.

You've heard this before, and it makes sense, right? So why haven't you done it?

Your Lifestyle Obstacles. Most people resist changing their lifestyle for two reasons.

Change is scary. Whether you realize it or not, your life is in a constant state of change. Though you cling to the familiar, it's a futile struggle. Change always wins.

The most consistent thing in life is change. Since you'll never escape it, you might as well channel it. It's time to make the change in your life purposeful and positive.

Lifestyle misconception. How many times have you heard the term 'healthy lifestyle' only to picture a health nut with celery sticks in one hand and tofu in the other? The truth is most people think that changing their lifestyle will be an extreme and unpleasant experience—and that's not true.

Improving your lifestyle does not mean swearing off chocolate or living in the gym. You don't have to eat wheat germ for lunch and you can still enjoy a nice plate of pasta. The key is moderation.

Making the Change. It's time to lose your 'all or nothing' mentality. Embrace simple, small changes that will add up to big improvements in your lifestyle. These are your main venues for change:

What You Eat. Let's face it; most of the foods you eat aren't the healthiest. Some are downright terrible (the burger and fries you had last week). While others are simply excessive (the snacks you eat while watching TV).

The solution to cleaning up your daily diet is NOT to go back on a 'diet'. In fact, I never want you to go on a 'diet' again. (Yes, you heard me right!) Instead, I want you to make permanent, healthy changes to your eating habits. Here are some practical examples:

- Choose salad over chips or fries
- Don't add butter to your food
- Eat fresh produce with every meal
- Purchase fat free dairy products
- Limit desserts to one or two per week
- Cut out mindless snacking
- Drink water, not soda

I don't expect you to eat a perfect diet every day of the week – that'd be ludicrous.

You should, however, make MORE healthy choices every day than unhealthy ones.

What You Do. Exercise is a huge component to a healthy lifestyle and quite frankly you're not getting enough of it. How often does an entire week go by without you ever lacing up your tennis shoes? Don't disregard the importance and power of a good workout.

Your new healthy lifestyle means exercising on most days of the week. This may seem tough, but I have the perfect solution – my training programs were created for busy people just like you who only have so much time to dedicate to exercise.

Here are simple ways to move more:

- Watch less TV
- Stretch stiff muscles every day
- Play at the park with the kids
- Go for a walk or jog
- Do some pushups every morning

While none of the above are meant as substitutes for your Fit Body Boot Camp workouts, they are great ways to become more active and to improve your lifestyle.

Your lifestyle is the balance of all the choices that you make regarding your body.

Swing the balance in your favor—make a majority of your choices health conscious.

So the next time you're in front of the mirror you won't worry about your weight.

You'll relish it.

The Top 7 Reasons to Exercise

Do you have reservations about the benefits of exercise? Here are 7 convincing reasons why you should lace up your workout shoes…

Reason #1: To Melt Fat Away

The most coveted side effect of exercise is, of course, fat burn. The combination of a challenging exercise routine and a balanced meal plan is the best known way to lose fat. Here's what losing fat feels like:

- Your pants become loose
- People around you begin to say that you look great
- A glance at yourself in the mirror makes you smile
- Your energy levels soar
- You feel amazing

Reason #2: To Alleviate Pain

Regular exercise is a great way to alleviate chronic muscle and joint pain. Persistent back pain can be lessened by strengthening your core and you'll protect yourself against injury. It amazes people when the chronic pain they've lived with for years begins to fade after starting a regular exercise program.

Reason #3: To Increase Lean Tissue

More muscle is good for many reasons. You see, muscle requires many more calories each day than fatty tissue. In fact, one pound of muscle burns 30-50 calories each day at rest—compared to a measly 9 calories per pound of fat.

When you exercise, your body composition will change to contain more lean tissue, thus resulting in extra calories burned while you sleep. What could be better than that?

Reason #4: To Stay Young

Tim D. Spector, a professor of genetic epidemiology at King's College in London, led a study on the effects of exercise on aging. The results were astounding. They found that exercise appears to slow the shriveling of the protective tips on bundles of genes inside cells (called telomeres), which means a slowing of the aging process.

"These data suggest that the act of exercising may actually protect the body against the aging process," said Spector.

Here's the study in a nutshell:

Telomeres cap the ends of chromosomes and every time a cell divides, the telomeres get shorter.

Once a telomere gets too short, that cell can no longer divide.

Aging occurs as more and more cells reach the end of their telomeres and die. This results in weakened muscles, skin wrinkles, loss of eyesight and hearing, organ failure, and slowed metal functioning.

The study analyzed the telomeres from the white bloods cells of twins over a 10-year period. Telomere length was used as a marker for the rate of biological aging.

It was found that the length of telomeres was directly related to that twin's activity level. "There was a gradient," Spector said. "As the amount of exercise increased, the telomere length increased."

People who did 100 minutes of weekly exercise had telomeres that looked like those from someone about 5-6 years younger than those who did 16 minutes of exercise each week.

People who did 3 hours of vigorous exercise each week had telomeres that looked like those from someone about 9 years younger.

Reason #5: To Prevent or Control Type 2 Diabetes

Regular exercise helps to stabilize blood sugar levels. This is something that people with type 2 diabetes, or at risk for type 2 diabetes gain substantial benefits from.

Exercise improves the body's use of insulin and the related weight loss improves insulin sensitivity. Of course patients with type 2 diabetes need to get guidelines from their doctor before starting an exercise program.

Reason #6: To Lower Blood Pressure and Cholesterol Levels

Exercise has shown to lower blood pressure and cholesterol levels for these two reasons:

Weak heart muscles pump little blood with lots of effort. By exercising you strengthen your heart muscles and train them to pump more blood with less effort. The stronger your heart is the less pressure will be exerted on your arteries.

Exercise increases HDL levels in some people—this means a decrease in your risk for heart disease. Other heart disease risk factors such as weight, diabetes, and high blood pressure all show improvement with regular exercise.

Reason #7: To Feel Great

The first thing clients tell me after starting an exercise program is how much better they feel.

Most didn't even realize how bad they felt. It is easy to get used to feeling sluggish, achy, and unmotivated.

Exercise boosts your energy levels and makes you feel amazing.

The quickest, easiest way to guarantee that you'll meet your fitness and weight loss goals is to work one-on-one with a qualified fitness professional. You'll be held accountable with your workouts and you'll be instructed properly and shown techniques and strategies that will expedite your results.

What are you waiting for? Lace up your shoes and get moving!

Your Reason

Your number one reason for exercise is unique to you.

Maybe you want to fit into a smaller pant size or lower your cholesterol.

Or maybe you just love how a good workout makes you feel.

Whatever your reason is, remind yourself of it often.

Write it down and place it where you will see it every day. It just may be the motivation you need.

Get Out Your Camera

Do you wish that you had more motivation to achieve your fitness goals?

Give yourself inspiration by taking a 'Before' picture.

That's right, put on your bathing suit and pose!

Next, place the picture in a place that you see often (on the refrigerator maybe?)

Now get to work on changing your body—imagine how great it will feel to replace your 'Before' picture with a stunning 'After' shot.

Here's an overview of this book. I have broken it down into 8 steps that will take you from where you are now to a place where you'll be living *The Fit Body Boot Camp Unstoppable Fat Loss Formula way.*

Step #1 What You Need to Know Before Ever Starting a "Diet" Program

Step #2 Foods That Burn Fat, Get You Fit, and Are Easy to Prepare

Step #3 Why You Should Never, Ever Eat These Foods - EVER

Step #4 Figuring Out When to Eat and How Much to Eat to Lose Maximum Fat

Step #5 How to Give Yourself a Proper Pantry Raid

Step #6 What to Eat When Eating Out

Step #7 How to Never Fail Again

Step #8 This Is Not a Diet - This Is a Lifestyle

Let's move on to Step #1...

CHAPTER TWO

Step #1 - What You Need To Know Before Ever Starting a "Diet" Program

There's one thing that will determine whether you end up at your goal weight or not.

One simple, powerful thing that you are in complete control of.

Your mind.

Before you begin your fat loss journey, it is vitally important that your mind is prepared for success.

Continue reading for tips and strategies to get into a fat burning mindset.

Do You Have the Stubborn Fat Blues?

Are you stuck in a body you aren't happy with?

Does it seem impossible for you to lose weight?

Do you get heavier each year?

So what do you do about the stubborn and seemingly permanent fat?

Sink into a depression?

Well, the easiest thing to do is to throw a pity party. Then before you know it your feelings of self-pity begin to snowball into a full blown case of the Stubborn Fat Blues.

How do you know if you have the Stubborn Fat Blues?

Your pants are tighter today than they were a year ago

You've tried to lose weight only to fail.

You feel trapped.

You're close to giving up on yourself.

If you can relate to any of the above statements then you have the Stubborn Fat Blues—quite an unpleasant condition to have.

Fortunately, there is a cure.

It all starts with your mind. The thing about the Stubborn Fat Blues is that it affects your mind more than anything else.

You see, your mental state is critical in determining your shape and size. When you focus on all of the things that you hate about your current body like the size of your thighs, the shape of your butt, or the way your belly looks then you're putting all of your energy towards the negative.

The more you think about how unhappy you are, the unhappier you will become.

Makes sense, right?

So instead of wallowing, use the following techniques to conquer the Stubborn Fat Blues:

Take it one battle at a time.

You may have 20, 50 or 100 pounds to lose before you reach your ideal weight—and that can be overwhelming. The truth is, weight loss like this won't happen overnight—it takes months of dedication. So, it's no wonder so many people simply give up.

Don't worry about winning the entire war today. Instead focus on conquering one battle at a time. Take it one meal at a time, and one day at a time. A healthy meal, a good workout, and you've won a battle. Remember, 100 pounds is broken down into 350,000 calories. Sure, that sounds like a lot, but all you have to do is focus on burning more calories than you take in today and in the end weight loss will be inevitable.

Use a trigger.

How many times throughout your day do you find yourself plagued with negative thoughts? *I'm too fat. I'll never look as good as I used to. I'm not attractive.* Yikes! Thoughts like these will ruin your chance at regaining your figure—they are total momentum killers.

Here's what I want you to do. Whenever a negative thought enters your mind instantly do the following:

Breathe out and squeeze your abs for 5 seconds – 3 times

Throw away any junk food within arms reach

Plan to exercise visit FBBC that day

Make negative thoughts a trigger to take positive action toward your goal—the results will amaze you.

See what you want.

If you have weight to lose, mirrors are a nightmare. Every lump and pouch seems to jump out with alarming illumination. And it doesn't help that most of us see things as worse than they really are.

When was the last time you closed your eyes and pictured the body you wished you had? It may sound hokey, but I'm serious. Your mind is very impressionable and when you bombard it with only the negative then you will be stuck on that image.

Take time each day to visualize your ideal body. Close your eyes and put yourself in that ideal body – feel what it feels like to be fit and attractive. This exercise is a powerful way to fixate your mind on your goal in a way that will leave you no room for failure.

Get serious.

Sooner or later you will decide that you are fed up with the Stubborn Fat Blues. You will decide that your health is important. You will decide that you deserve to look great. And you will do what it takes to achieve amazing results.

The best way to ensure that your motivation stays strong—and that your goal is met—is to get into your local Fit Body Boot Camp location for support and for fat burning workouts.

Together we will identify your goals, find workout programs that you enjoy and create a routine that works with your schedule. It's that simple.

Then you can say goodbye to the Stubborn Fat Blues—forever!

The Blame Game

Whose fault is it that you're out of shape?

If you go by what you hear in diet ads then you believe that it's anyone's fault but yours.

The big diet companies think that if they put the blame on you then you wouldn't buy their bogus pills. So they put the blame on your cortisol levels, your modern diet (i.e. fast food), or your busy schedule instead of where it belongs—which is squarely on your shoulders.

Sure, you have obstacles that get in your way – your schedule, your job, your kids, the weather, your knee injury from college…but ultimately you have the body that you accept.

I'm going to repeat that so it will really sink in.

You have the body that you accept…But you can change it.

Embracing the blame for your current weight is not a bad thing – it's empowering.

Think about it. If it really wasn't your fault, if it really was due to a long list of variables that you have zero control over, then you'd be stuck. You'd have no way to change.

The Secret Behind 'Before and After' Pictures

Allow me to pull back the curtain for you on something that the diet industry doesn't want you to know. You've seen countless before and after pictures documenting weight loss as a result of a diet product. Well, there is more involved than just the diet product. No one can take a simple product and presto have the perfect before and after picture. There is much more involved that the diet industry doesn't share.

Look into the eyes of any person in their before picture and you'll see that they are disturbed. The body they have is no longer in sync with the body they can accept.

They changed the body that they accept.

Now look into their eyes in the after picture – see the sweet satisfaction? They now own the body that they decided they could accept; and what a great feeling that is.

Your Time To Transform

Whether you realize it or not, you already posses everything you need to transform your body, but it all starts with taking responsibility for the body that you have today. You have your current body because until this moment you've been OK with it.

Oh sure you aren't thrilled with it, and you even talk about losing weight and getting fit, but you haven't changed what you'll accept. Here's how to transform your body in 3 steps:

Step One: Get Disturbed

You've heard it said that *emotion creates motion*. This is essential when it comes to losing weight. Just like those folks in the before pictures, to transform your body you must first decide that you can't live another day in the body you currently have.

It's time to get your emotions stirred up. Make a list of all the reasons that you *must* lose weight and get fit. Get disturbed!

Step Two: Get Focused

Without clarity it's very hard to get where you want to go. Now that you're disturbed with the body you have, it's time to decide what the body you can accept looks like.

I want you to think in concrete and specific terms. Just like the captions under those before and after pictures—"Suzy lost 25 lbs," "Mike lost 8 inches from his waist," "Jenny went from a size 18 to a size 6."

Get a clear picture in your mind of what you'll look like in *your* after picture and visualize what the caption will read.

Step Three: Get Moving

The time spent between your inspiration (now) and your action determines whether you will succeed or fail. Don't allow yourself to get stuck between inspiration and action—there is always *something* that you can do right now.

Don't you agree that you'll be happier living life in a fit, healthy, and attractive body, rather than the body you have today? Of course you'll be happier.

Fit Body Boot Camp has helped scores of clients just like you finally lose their unwanted weight.

We are here to take you from your before picture to your after picture; however, you need to bring something to the table – you need to make up your mind about what you'll accept of yourself.

What will you accept?

_____

Do You Have What it Takes to Get the Body of Your Dreams?

For many, the summer months bring with them a harsh reminder of unmet fitness goals.

While the toned men and slender women of the world put on their skin-tastic summer gear and proudly put themselves on display, those with jiggles and dimples would rather opt for a cover up and hang out under an umbrella.

So why haven't you met your fitness goals?

Why must you go through another agonizing summer, turning your head as you pass by a dozen magazines showcasing skinny celebrities in bikinis? You should be enjoying your summer days without wondering which pair of shorts covers the most.

The truth is that anyone can get the body of their dreams…even you. And wouldn't it feel great to put on your bathing suit without bracing yourself before looking in the mirror?

You can turn your fitness dreams into reality—read on for the three things you need to begin achieving amazing results.

Your Mind

You may be wondering what your mind has to do with getting your body into great shape. In a single word, your mind has *everything* to do with getting the body of your dreams. Your mind will single handedly make or break your success.

How? Well, your mind works hard to reinforce the beliefs that you hold about yourself. If you think of yourself as a fat person, or an out-of-shape person, or just an average person then your subconscious mind will do everything in its power to keep you that way.

It's like self-sabotage.

However, if you begin to think of yourself as fit, healthy and attractive, then your mind will do everything it can to make your belief a reality.

*Take time everyday to visualize your new body and to focus on your goals.

Your Plan

Everyone who successfully sets out to lose body fat and achieve results does so by implementing a plan. Your plan is crucial to your success, picture it as a guiding map needed to find a new destination. Without it you are lost.

Here are the two major parts to your plan:

1. Diet: They say you are what you eat, and that is never truer than while losing weight. Cut junk food from your diet and stick with fresh healthy foods instead. Eat small meals throughout the day containing protein, good fibrous carbohydrates, and minimal fat.

2. Exercise: Yes, you will have to break a sweat, but the good news is once you make exercise a habit you will likely find it to be enjoyable – In fact, I know you will. It is important that you make exercise a part of your lifestyle and not something that you do on random occasions. For maximal results exercise 4-5 times each week doing both cardiovascular and resistance training.

*Stick with your healthy eating plan and exercise routine—these are the building blocks to your success.

Your Determination

Determination is the one thing that will guarantee that you will lose weight, tone your body, and feel better than ever. You have to want it—that's it. Thinking about it is not enough. Now it's time for action!

You have to want your dream body…

- *more* than you want that burger and fries.

- *more* than you want to skip your workout.

- *more* than you want that chocolate cookie.

- *more* than you want to sit on the couch.

The shape and size of your body is in your hands, and your hands only. I believe that you possess the kind of determination that it takes to change your body—you simply need to dig down deep enough within yourself to find it.

Fuel your fire by building a network of support in your life. Enlist friends, family, and loved ones to encourage your efforts and to keep tabs on your progress. In fact, we would love to be a key player in your network of support—become a part of the Fit Body Boot Camp Facebook fan page or don't hesitate to email or call us and get onboard with the best fitness program. Fitness is our passion and we can help make it yours too!

*Surround yourself with support and <u>don't give up</u>.

We get excited when talking about getting you the body of your dreams—this is what we do everyday for our clients. Making the decision to transform your body is something to celebrate.

The Power of Your Self-Image

How will you harness your potential to create the very best you?

I recommend using the teachings of Dr. Maxwell Maltz in his legendary book *The New Psycho-Cybernetics.*

Dr. Maltz created the original science of self-improvement and success, so who better to turn to when you're ready to take your life to another level. His teachings have stood the test of time.

Take the following and get all that you want:

Use Your Imagination

If you thought that imaginations were only valued in preschool, think again. One of the key points in *The New Psycho-Cybernetics* is the technique of using your imagination to reprogram and manage your self-image.

You may have been exposed to self improvement strategies that tell you to 'act as if' or to 'fake it till you make it.' Those typically don't work because your self image is still the same.

According to Dr. Maltz, your self-image is the key to changing your actions and habits. If you want to lose 50 pounds you first have to think of yourself as someone 50 pounds lighter.

Spend time in your imagination. See yourself 50 pounds lighter. Experience a day in your life at this slimmed down size. Imagine everything down to the smallest detail.

According to Dr. Maltz, this imagination time will begin to change your self-image to that of a person 50 pounds lighter and your actions and habits will fall into place.

Reject Negative Thoughts

Negative thoughts will undoubtedly arise as you use your imagination to see your ideal self.

"I'm not really going to lose 50 pounds." "I've tried losing weight before and it never works. I'm always going to be overweight." "This imagination stuff is bogus. It won't work for me."

Dr. Maltz says that the instant you receive a negative thought simply dismiss it. Don't spend any time on it at all.

The quicker that you dismiss negative thoughts, the less impact they will have on your self-image. Also you'll find that fewer and fewer negative thoughts arise once you get into the habit of dismissal.

Be Nostalgic For The Future

It's so easy to be nostalgic for the past especially when you only remember the good stuff. But what good does it do for you to wish for things that are long gone?

Dr. Maltz recommends developing nostalgia for the future.

In your imagination you've already lost the 50 pounds, so start pining for the future! Your self-image will lock onto that picture and your nostalgic feelings will fuel the fire.

I'm The Kind Of Person That...

What kind of person are you?

I'm the kind of person that loves sweets.

I'm the kind of person that hates exercise.

I'm the kind of person that can't lose weight.

OR

I'm the kind of person that eats fresh and healthy food.

I'm the kind of person that keeps fit.

I'm the kind of person that maintains an ideal body weight.

Your self-image will fulfill any label that you put on yourself. The power is all in your hands.

What kind of a person do you want to be?

_____

Find Reward in The Process

Have you noticed a pattern?

You'll spend a couple of weeks eating clean, exercising and losing weight, but then the pendulum swings and you spend the next week or two indulging in your old unhealthy habits.

After enough chubby days you'll get back to your clean habits and so the yo-yo continues.

It's time to stop this vicious cycle that never brings you all the way to your goal, keeping you comfortable enough, yet frustrated.

The good news is that your yo-yo days could be quickly and permanently turned off with this simple mindset change.

Find your reward in the process, not in the results.

When it comes to weight loss, we've been brainwashed to focus all of our efforts on the "results". Your desired result is the ideal body that you dream to have – it's your reason for passing on dessert and the image you hold in your mind as you toil through burpees and mountain climbers.

News flash: If you only find reward in the results, you're likely to fail.

What?!?

Think about it. Results are abstract.

Oh sure, you can picture it in your mind with crystal clarity but what reach does that image have on you when you're lured into the drive thru?

Let's face it—future results are easy to lose focus on.

The Process: this is the act of working toward your goal – your meal plan, your exercise routine, and your healthy life style choices.

If you had a map of where you are today (blue dot) and where you'll be when you reach your goal (red dot) the process is that black line connecting the two.

When all you're focused on to reinforce your journey is the promise of results, it's easy to wind up lost.

Finding Reward in the Process: Make a new habit of feeling rewarded after every day on your chosen path.

Completing your diet and exercise each day needs to become its own reward. Look down and applaud yourself for each step forward.

When you find reward in the process, the results will take care of themselves.

Getting Past Mental Roadblocks

Most people wait around for motivation to strike them like a lightning bolt.

Well, I've got news: motivation isn't something that happens to you—it's something that you create for yourself.

If you don't feel motivated to achieve your goals, it is likely due to mental roadblocks that hold you hostage.

Read the following **21 Mindset Tips** and prepare your mind for success.

Success comes first in the mind, so visualize yourself accomplishing your goals.

Remember, you are the only person who can hold you back.

Forgive yourself and love yourself despite past failures.

Decide what is important in your life and focus on that.

Conquer each negative thought the moment it enters your mind, when it is weakest.

Give up the idea that things won't go right unless you worry about them.

If you bring the body of your dreams to the point of resolve, then you'll soon be living in it.

Look towards your future. If you believe the best is yet to come then it will be.

You become what you think about most.

The margin between success and failure is very small and easily bridged by determination.

Start your day by accomplishing your hardest task first.

Set small attainable goals, rather than one monumental goal.

Convince yourself that exercise is fun, and it will be.

Know your big reason why.

Create a motivating play list of songs to use as the sound track to your workout sessions.

Every decision you make leads you either closer toward achieving your goal or farther from it.

If you think you're a fat person, then you'll stay fat. If you think you're fit, then you soon will be.

Once you've set your goal, your attitude either pushes you toward accomplishment or failure.

If you don't know exactly where you want to go, you will likely end up someplace else.

You can have the body of your dreams, but first you must give up the belief that you can't.

You can only have two things in life: excuses or results.

Can You Change in a Single Moment?

Change is a curious thing. In most areas of life you dread it, yet in others you pine for it.

You're told that change is hard, that it takes time. You're also told that change is the most consistent thing you'll encounter. You wonder how to make lasting changes that will improve your life.

I'm here to argue that change can happen in an instant.

I know this goes against mainstream belief. Most people believe that change has to be worked at for months or even years. We expect to try and fail numerous times before we ultimately give up or succeed.

Think about it—how many people do you know who struggle with their weight? They want to make a healthy change by getting in shape, but the change never seems to take hold.

Is there something in your life that you want to change? Do you have weight to lose? Do you have high blood pressure, high cholesterol, or a pair of pants that you wish you could fit into?

What is preventing you from making a positive change in your life?

According to professional speaker and author, Anthony Robbins, it's the getting ready to change that takes time. In the end there's an instant when the change occurs. Robbins goes on to outline three specific beliefs that you must have in order to instantly create a lasting change.

Belief #1: Something **<u>must</u>** change.

Do you kind of want to get into shape or do you absolutely have to lose the weight? Does dropping a few pounds sound nice or is living another day in your current body simply out of the question? In order to make a lasting change you must be convinced that the time is right.

Belief #2: <u>I</u> must change it.

It is vital that you take full responsibility in making the change. Sure others may assist you, but in the end you are the one who is going to make it happen. You have to want this change enough to make it your personal mission—no one else will do it for you.

Belief #3: I **<u>can</u>** change it.

Don't let past failures get in your way. The truth is that you can do amazing things when you put your mind to it. Believe that you are capable of losing weight or making any other positive change in your life.

Why do most people fail to make lasting change? They leave it up to willpower. This works for awhile, but you'll always revert back to what's comfortable. The solution?

Change what you're comfortable with.

You've probably heard that humans are motivated by two things: 1) to avoid pain and 2) to gain pleasure. When you want to change a behavior pattern the key is to associate pain with the behavior that you don't want and pleasure with the behavior that you do want.

You know that you want to lose weight and that to do so you need to quit eating comfort food late at night. You also know that you need to start exercising on a regular basis. Up until this point your brain is trained to associate pleasure with eating comfort food late at night and to associate pain with exercise.

It's time to retrain your brain to feel good about exercise and to feel bad about eating late at night. Think about all of the negative things about being overweight and connect these unpleasant thoughts to your late night snack. Now think about all of the wonderful things about being in shape and connect these pleasant thoughts to exercise.

You are capable of making a big change in your life.

Remember, change can happen in an instant.

It's Your Turn

Think for a moment of that huge accomplishment that you haven't made.

Maybe it's a weight loss goal that you've had for years.

Maybe it's something completely unrelated to your weight.

What's holding you back?

Are you afraid you'll fail?

The fear of failure is a powerful thing. No one likes to fail, and repeat failure is even worse. So what can you do to conquer it?

Realize that failure isn't the worst outcome. Not trying is.

You only fail when you decide to give up. Get up and try again!

Are you afraid you'll succeed?

You may not realize it, but most people fear success. Success means change and change can be scary. It is important that you embrace the idea of success and ditch any negative self-talk.

Close your eyes and picture yourself accomplishing your goal. What will that accomplishment do for your life? List the benefits you'll enjoy.

Spend a few minutes each day visualizing yourself accomplishing your goal. How great does it feel? Savor those victorious emotions and use them to drive your motivation.

It's your turn to accomplish something huge.

5 Simple Steps for Achieving Any Goal

If you're not happy with your body then your workouts have lost focus.

What is your immediate goal?

If you don't have a ready answer then chances are good that your motivation is low and it has resulted in a lack of results.

I know from firsthand experience that operating without a goal will get you nowhere. Sure, you may still be exercising regularly and eating mindfully but without that concrete goal your efforts will yield little results.

1. Setting your goal

You want to be in "better shape" but that's so vague. Dig deeper.

What specifically do you wish you had now that you don't?

To drop 3 dress sizes.

To lose 2 inches of arm fat jiggle.

To melt 4 inches from your waist.

To be able to run 3 miles without stopping.

2. Define your timeline

Now that you've determined exactly what part of your body isn't up to par, tie that goal in with a specific timeline. When you have a timeline to measure your progress against, you'll find that achieving your goal becomes an easier process.

To drop 3 dress sizes by August 20th vacation.

To lose 2 inches of arm fat jiggle by October 13th wedding.

To melt 4 inches from your waist by July 7th pool party.

To be able to run 3 miles without stopping by June 16th city 5k.

3. Name your prize

It's time to take your motivation to the next level. Now that your specific goal is set and your timeline is clearly defined, let's add a prize that you'll receive once you've accomplished your goal. This prize shouldn't be anything related to your unhealthy habits – so no junk food or extra large meals. Make the prize an item that will reinforce your slimmer body, like a nice piece of clothing.

A couple new outfits for your August vacation.

A sleeveless dress for the October wedding.

A new swimsuit for your July pool party.

A new pair of running shoes for your June 5k.

4. Picture it

You know what you want, when you want it by, and the reward you'll get by achieving it. Now spend time picturing your end goal. Find a comfortable, quiet corner, close your eyes and see a mental movie – starring yourself – enjoying your reward with your new and improved body. Play your mental success movie several times throughout the day.

See yourself enjoying an afternoon of your vacation, wearing your new clothes with confidence.

Imagine how you'll feel walking down the aisle baring your toned arms.

See yourself lounging by the pool in your swimsuit, carefree and happy.

Imagine the feeling of accomplishment you'll feel as you cross the finish line.

5. Recipe for success

The steps that you've taken above have prepared you to mentally take on the challenge of motivating yourself through this transformation process. All that remains is a solid exercise and nutrition plan to push you through to your new body.

How to Achieve Any Goal

Do you have unmet goals?

You aren't alone. In fact, many people live with unfulfilled aspirations and the self-help industry is booming as a result.

Unfortunately, many widely used self-help techniques fail to deliver results.

Case in point: You've probably heard of the "Yale Goal Study" in which researchers were said to have interviewed the graduating Yale seniors in 1953, asking whether or not the students had written down specific goals that they wanted to achieve.

Then 20 years down the road the researchers looked up each student and discovered that the 3% of the class who had written down their goals had accumulated more personal wealth than the other 97% combined.

Very compelling story, but complete fiction.

The "Yale Goal Study" never happened, though motivational speakers and self-help books have quoted it for years.

Best selling author and psychologist Richard Wiseman went on a mission to craft a no-nonsense response to the bogus self-help techniques. Using a diverse range of scientific data he uncovered a proven approach to achieve any goal.

The following 5 successful techniques (Do This) and 5 unsuccessful techniques (Not That) are from Wiseman's book, *59 Seconds Change Your Life in Under a Minute*.

Do This: Make a Step-by-Step Plan.

If you are serious about achieving your goal, then you need to create a step-by-step plan on how to do it.

Successful goal-achievers break down their overall goal into sub-goals. Each sub-goal needs to be concrete, measurable and time-based.

Not That: Motivate yourself by focusing on someone that you admire.

Studies show that focusing on someone you admire is not a strong enough motivator to see you through your goal.

Do This: Tell Other People About Your Goal.

How badly do you want to achieve your goal? If you want it bad enough, you'll tell your friends and family.

This technique works on two levels. First, you've put yourself on the spot by letting the world in on your goal, so it's all-eyes-on-you. Failure would be public. Second, your friends and family are there to offer support and encouragement. Don't underestimate the psychological power of having someone in your corner.

Not That: Think about the bad things.

When you focus on the negative it becomes your reality.

Do This: Focus on the Good Things When Achieving Your Goal.

Remind yourself of the benefits associated with achieving your goal.

Make a checklist of how life will be better once you have achieved your aim. This gets your focus on a positive future, one that's worth the effort.

Not That: Try to suppress unhelpful thoughts.

Rather than trying to erase that image of chocolate cake from your mind, learn to deal with the reality of temptation head-on.

Do This: Reward Your Progress.

Studies show that attaching rewards to each of your sub-goals encourages success.

Your rewards should never conflict with your major goal. When aiming to lose weight, never use food as a reward.

Not That: Rely on willpower.

Willpower alone rarely gets anyone to their goal.

Do This: Record Your Progress.

Make your plans, progress, benefits, and rewards concrete by expressing them in writing.

Use a hand-written journal, your computer or a bulletin board to chart your progress. This process is priceless for maintaining motivation.

Not That: Fantasize about life after achieving your goal.

Daydreaming is fun, but simply fantasizing about your new life will not make it a reality.

Now is your time to get into the best shape of your life.

Is your goal SMART?

Do you know why you exercise? Is it to lose weight? Is it to lower your blood pressure or cholesterol? Is it to shrink your waist? Is it to pick up a bag of groceries with more ease?

The first step toward getting the body of your dreams is to set a goal. This simple act, when done correctly, will instantly calm your frustrations and fill you with hope.

Here's how to make your goals **SMART**.

Specific: Ask yourself questions like: How many inches do I want to lose? What pant size do I want to be? Be painstakingly specific with yourself. It has been proven that the more specific your goal is the more likely you are to achieve it.

Measurable: You've got to be able to measure your results. It could be in pounds or body fat percentage or inches. It could even be fitting into a particular pair of pants that you haven't worn in years. The key is that you need to be able to physically measure your progress.

Attainable: If you have 50 pounds to lose it won't all come off in one month. Setting unattainable goals simply sets you up for failure. If you have a major fat loss goal then break it down into small attainable goals. As you achieve each smaller goals you will reinforce your progress and ultimately can attain any desired goal.

Realistic: This step is all about knowing yourself. What type of program would you realistically stick with? If you despise running then don't base your weight loss program on 6AM jogs. Look honestly at your abilities, but don't underestimate yourself either. You'll need to push yourself to achieve your goal.

Timely: Every great goal is set on a timeline. Keeping the above steps in mind, give yourself an exact date and time that your goal needs to be accomplished by.

Now it's time to get to work. Write down your **SMART** goal and place it somewhere that you see often then tell three people of importance in your life about your goal.

Have the focus and the drive to pursue your **SMART** goal.

Find Your Motivation

Motivation comes from having a goal. What is your goal? Why do you want to get into great shape?

Take a minute to really uncover the reason that you want to lose the weight. Don't say something vague like you want to *'Be thinner'* or *'Look more attractive.'*

Dig deeper – there is a very specific motivator in your life you simply need to uncover it.

Here are some possible motivators...

I want to have more energy to keep up with the kids.

I want to improve my health through weight loss to extend and improve my life.

I want to lose 15 pounds before my vacation.

I want to restore my confidence to wear sleeveless shirts.

I want to regain my figure to impress and attract my significant other.

Why Aren't You Motivated?

A good dose of motivation can change your life almost overnight.

The best part of my job is seeing clients achieve amazing results. Whether they drop a few sizes, lose baby weight, get off their blood pressure meds, or shrink their waist; the excitement is always contagious.

There really isn't a clear way to describe the euphoria that settles in once you've realized your fitness goal. You have to experience it.

Though each successful client is unique with different goals, one element unites them.

They are all highly motivated.

You see, I am in a unique position. I know how to get you into great shape. I can coach you through a 50 pound weight loss. I can guide you to a healthier body. I can even train you into a toned athlete.

But there is one catch.

You'll need to be motivated.

See, saying that you want to get into great shape isn't enough. You need motivation—and that's just half of the equation. The other part (and the most important) is **ACTION**.

Nothing happens until you take *action*.

You can want it, think about it, mull it over, ponder it, plan it, and then re-plan it. But nothing happens until you take action.

While I may not know your story—it's probably safe to assume that you are dissatisfied with your body and know that you can improve your fitness level. You want to look better, have more energy, experience fewer aches and pains, and enjoy sweet satisfaction as you achieve your goals once and for all.

I know that all of my successful clients were once in your shoes. They wanted to change their bodies. They felt urgency. And then they did what most fail to do. They took action and contacted me.

But there is more to it than that. They then committed to a program, did the exercise, stuck to their diet, and met their goals. There's nothing more gratifying than getting back into those jeans that now sit in the back of your closet.

Those that take massive action get massive rewards. And those that simply talk about losing weight will continue to put weight on, pound after pound. I hate to put it that way, but it's the truth.

So what do you want?

To drop 20 pounds

To feel younger

To look better in your birthday suit

How bad do you want it? How much motivation do you have? Enough to take MASSIVE ACTION?

The rewards are great IF you do.

Picture This

Having trouble with motivation? Try this technique:

Go through your photo albums and find a picture of yourself in your best shape ever. It may be a photo from your college or even high school days.

Now go through your photos and find a picture of yourself in your worst shape ever. You may have to go through old shoe boxes of photos, since this photo may not have made it into your photo albums.

Place the two photos side by side. You at your fittest; you at your fattest. Study the photos. Remember what it felt like to be in great shape. Remember what it felt like to be in terrible shape (you may be living that right now).

Make a decision. Do you want to continue living your life in bad shape? Or will you shake off past failures and do what it takes to achieve the body you once had?

Bring your photos in to your local Fit Body Boot Camp location and get ready to take **ACTION**.

The Missing Link for Motivation

If you've ever wished that you were more motivated to experience life at your full potential then this is for you.

Most of us set goals and work hard only to find our motivation fizzle out after a couple of weeks. But there are little tricks that will help you harness the power of your mind and propel you toward achieving your goal.

The Two Motivators

When you narrow it down, you're motivated by two simple things:

To avoid pain (fear of failure)

To gain pleasure (promise of reward)

You are naturally geared toward one of these motivators.

To figure out which, think of the last time you accomplished a task and then ask yourself the following: While doing the task were you thinking about what would happen if you failed to finish, or were you thinking about what you would gain when you finished?

Take note as to which motivator works for you – fear of failure, or promise of reward.

Set Your Goal: The first step towards unstoppable motivation is to determine your goal. You know you're unhappy with your body, but what exactly do you want to change? Why is it important to you?

Perhaps you can relate to one of the following goals:

You need to lose weight for your health. Your doctor scared you straight or maybe you've had a recent health problem that landed you in the hospital.

Your goal is to move away from the pain of sickness.

You want to look and feel incredible. You've always wanted to feel vibrant and attractive. The idea of having more energy really excites you.

Your goal is to move toward the pleasure and reward of a fit body.

You're worried about your kids. They don't eat enough vegetables, they drink more soda pop than water, and they play video games constantly. You have decided to model a healthier lifestyle and to encourage your kids to participate.

Your goal is to move away from the risks of a sedentary lifestyle and to propel your kids toward a healthy future.

Train Your Mind for Weight Loss: With your clear and important goal in mind, let's take a few minutes to train your mind to achieve it. You know that weight loss comes as a result of eating right and regular challenging exercise, so let's use your mind to conquer both.

Eating Right: Use this exercise to distance yourself from the self-sabotaging foods you really wish you didn't eat and to naturally begin selecting healthy foods.

Take a moment to review your current eating habits. Identify the foods that you should stop eating (hint: sweets, anything fried, refined carbohydrates, sugary drinks). Identify the worst food that you eat regularly but know you shouldn't.

Now imagine the healthy foods that you should eat (hint: vegetables, fruits, whole grains, lean protein). Identify the healthiest food that you know you should eat regularly.

Now with the image of these two foods in mind, find a quiet place and do the following exercise (seriously this stuff works):

Draw up the image of your unhealthy food item. This image will likely be quite vivid, with smell, taste and bright color. In your mind, fade this picture to black and white and distance the image until it is dull, fuzzy and remote.

Draw up the image of your healthy food item. This image will likely be fuzzy and faded. In your mind, bring this picture to life with smell, taste, sound and bright color.

Regular Exercise: This technique can be applied in a way that encourages you to crave exercise rather than avoid it.

Take a moment to imagine how you feel *after* a great workout (notice the emphasis on the word *after*). Remember the physical satisfaction as well as the sweet feeling of accomplishment.

Now bring to your mind the aspects of exercise that you dislike. What is your biggest reason for avoiding exercise? Are you too tired? Do you not have enough time? Is physical exertion too much of a hassle? Pinpoint your greatest complaint about exercise.

Now with the image of these two aspects of exercise in mind, find a quiet place and do the following exercise:

Draw up the image of your exercise complaint. The image is likely to be clear and accompanied by the sounds, smells, and sensations. In your mind, fade this picture to black and white and distance the image until it is dull, fuzzy, and remote.

Draw up the image of the wonderful feeling you have after accomplishing a great workout. Magnify this image in your mind. Fixate on how you feel physically, mentally, and emotionally. View the experience in bright colors and add a sound track of inspirational music.

Why It Works: If this was your first experience with training your mind (also called Neuro-Linguistic Programming, or NLP) it may have felt a little odd. Many of the world's top achievers regularly use techniques like these to accomplish astounding goals.

The techniques above work because they train your mind to bring your behavior in line with your values. Think about it, you value health, you desire to be fit and attractive, and you want to instill healthy habits in your kids.

These techniques encourage you to avoid self-sabotage and to make choices that line up with what you truly value.

The Rocking Chair Test

Need another boost of motivation? Anthony Robbins uses this Rocking Chair Test to propel his students to action.

Imagine yourself at 90 years old, sitting in a rocking chair and looking back over your life.

Imagine that you never accomplished the goals that are important to you. Feel the pain of loss and regret.

Now imagine that you did accomplish these important goals. Feel the pleasure of success and accomplishment.

Which scenario do you want to experience when you are 90?

Your Ideal You

Take a moment and imagine your 'ideal *you*'.

What does the 'ideal *you*' look like?

How does the 'ideal *you*' spend their time?

Who would the 'ideal *you*' spend time with?

What would the 'ideal *you*' accomplish?

The distance between you and your 'ideal *you*' is created by laziness.

When faced with decisions, big or small, do what your 'ideal *you*' would do, rather than taking the easy way out.

(I'm pretty sure that your 'ideal *you*' is a client of Fit Body Boot Camp… ☺)

_____

Now that your mind is primed and ready for success, let's move on to Step #2…

CHAPTER THREE

Step #2 - Foods That Burn Fat, Get You Fit, and Are Easy to Prepare

In the fitness industry it's a well know fact that the shape of your body is due 80% to the foods you choose to eat and only 20% due to the exercise you perform.

80% of what your body looks like is <u>because of what you eat</u>.

What you eat seriously matters!

If you want to be lean and free from excess body fat then you must train yourself to eat the right foods.

Many foods are labeled as "healthy" even though they lead to weight gain.

In this section you will learn exactly which foods to eat and which to avoid.

The Right Foods

Choosing the right foods is easier than you'd think.

Close your eyes and imagine that you're a caveman. You can picture him. Long hair, rippling muscles, and raw strength. He has no grocery store or fast food joint at his disposal. So what did he eat?

Plants and Animals.

These two categories comprised most of his diet – and it should yours too.

Your goal should be to eat plants and animals as 80% or more of your diet and the remaining 20% or less should be nuts, legumes, and some whole grains.

Simple, right?

Eat Clean to Be Lean

Many people want to lose weight and maybe you are one who has been trying hard for months and hasn't had much success.

You've heard fitness people refer to 'eating clean' but what does that really mean?

The labels on hundreds of different food items proclaim to be 'healthy' but can you trust labels? There are so many misconceptions when it comes to what constitutes as clean eating.

What are you eating wrong?

Let's dispel the myths and outline your simple, straightforward 3-step guide to eating clean and start watching the pounds melt off.

Step One: Steer Clear of Packaged Foods

Your worst enemy in the fight against weight gain is packaged foods. Yes, even those packages that are described as 'healthy'.

Think of packaged food in these 3 categories:

Sweets: Cookies, brownies, muffins, cupcakes, donuts, candy, and desserts. These packaged items are laced with sugar and bad fats, and lack any viable nutrient that your body actually needs. All the empty calories from these items will end up deposited on your waist and hips as stubborn fat.

There's never a good reason to eat these so-called foods.

Processed Grains: Crackers, breads, cereal, chips, instant oatmeal, energy bars, and popcorn This category is tricky because many of the packages are labeled as 'heart healthy' or 'low fat'. The reality is that packaged, processed grains contain sugar and more carbohydrates than you need while striving to lose weight.

If you have a weight loss goal then stay away from processed grains.

Whole Grains: Brown rice, wild rice, whole oats, sprouted grain pasta, and sprouted grain bread. Here's a category of packaged foods that you are able to include in your clean diet. You don't, however, have a free pass to eat as much of these items as you'd like. Whole grains, while healthy and acceptable, are very calorie-dense. This means that a little bit goes a long way.

Eat whole grains in moderation in order to meet your weight loss goals.

Step Two: Fill Up on Fresh Foods

Fresh vegetables and fruits are a huge part of your clean diet.

The nutrients and fiber found in these natural food items are vitally important for your weight loss journey and your overall health.

Eat a variety of fruits and vegetables in all shapes, sizes, and colors.

The only ones that you need to limit are vegetables that are high in starch, such as potatoes and corn, and fruits that are very high in sugar, like melons.

Step Three: Get Plenty of Protein

The cornerstone of your clean diet should be lean protein.

Great examples are chicken breast, albacore tuna, lean ground turkey, white fish fillet, whole beans, tempeh, and egg whites.

Protein is what holds your clean eating plan together, for two reasons:

Protein satiates your hunger, keeping you full and keeping your blood sugar stable. This eliminates false hunger and prevents unnecessary snacking.

Protein helps to grow and maintain your muscle mass, which increases your resting metabolism. This means that your body will be naturally leaner.

Making the Healthy Choice

As a rule of thumb ignore the bold claims on food packaging—the information you really need is listed on the nutrition label. Finding healthy food is simple when you use the following guidelines.

Eat Fresh: The healthiest food in the world is fresh, unprocessed whole foods. This includes fresh vegetables and fruit, whole grains and legumes, and raw seeds and nuts. These fresh foods supply your body with vitamins, minerals, and enzymes that are priceless to your health. When it comes to meat, poultry, and dairy choose products that are grass fed and hormone and antibiotic free.

Set Limits: Let's be honest. Just because something is edible doesn't mean you should eat it. A key to healthy eating is to identify which items to limit or even eliminate from your diet.

Cholesterol. The American Heart Association recommends that you limit your intake of cholesterol from food to less than 300 milligrams per day.

Saturated Fat. Your intake of saturated fat should be less than 7% of your total daily calories.

Trans Fat. It is recommended that you either eliminate trans fat from your diet or keep it under 1% of your total daily calories.

Sugar. Most of us consume way more sugar than we should. Make a habit of checking the ingredient list of the foods you eat. If sugar is the first listed ingredient then you know that item is packed with sugar.

Look at the whole picture: A healthy diet consists of taking in a combination of fats, carbohydrates, fiber, protein, vitamins, and minerals each day. Remember, eating too much of even healthy foods can lead to weight gain. All of the foods that you eat should fit together to form a well-balanced, calorie controlled diet.

The bottom line is that you should eat to live not live to eat. Your body will thank you for it.

The Missing Link to Optimal Health

Do you rarely get sick, have no need for prescription meds, and can't remember the last time you had to visit the doctor?

If you answered no to the above questions then you are likely suffering from nutritional deficiencies.

It's hard to know exactly what to eat for optimal health, especially since everyone has a different opinion.

Even when you make every effort to eat healthy, your diet almost always lacks important nutrients.

In Victoria Boutenko's book, *Green For Life,* she set out in search of the perfect human diet. She immersed herself in nutrition research and discovered a very interesting observation.

The Chimpanzee Connection: Chimpanzees and humans are more closely related than any other animal species. In fact, research shows that we share 99.4% of our DNA sequence with our chimpanzee friends.

Why is this significant? Chimpanzees are in far better physical shape than humans and possess strong natural immunity to cancer and other fatal -- and quite common -- human illnesses.

Victoria's research all pointed to the chimpanzee diet as the reason for their superior health. Chimps and humans have vastly different eating habits.

It's All About The Greens: While humans enjoy pizza and hamburgers, chimps eat a diet extremely high in dark leafy greens -- an item that hardly exists in the human world.

Victoria then turned her focus on dark leafy greens. What she discovered was a super-food packed with extremely high levels of nutrients. Here are five amazing facts about greens:

1. Greens are packed with amino acids (AKA protein).

I'll bet you didn't know that dark leafy greens are a legitimate source of protein. It's true!

Protein molecules are made of a chain of amino acids. When you consume protein from chicken, you're getting chains of amino acids that have already been assembled into a complex protein.

When you eat dark leafy greens you are getting a plethora of individual amino acids. Your body then takes these amino acids and assembles it into complex protein chains.

2. Greens give you lots of insoluble fiber (like a sponge).

You know fiber is important, but did you realize that fiber is needed to rid your body of toxins? Insoluble fiber is extra special since it is built like tiny sponges that each absorbs several times more toxins than its own volume.

Check out just a few of the many benefits of fiber:

* Fiber reduces cholesterol

* Fiber prevents and reduces the risk of cancer

* Fiber lessens risk of diabetes and improves existing diabetes

* Fiber helps shed unwanted pounds and prevents overeating

3. Greens promote bodily homeostasis...necessary for optimal health.

Homeostasis is the physiological process that regulates all substances in your body at ideal levels for optimal health. It is a very complex process, one that your body is constantly working towards.

In order for your body to achieve homeostasis it needs an abundance of vitamins, amino acids, carbohydrates, essential fatty acids, and minerals. Greens are a super provider of all of the above.

4. Greens are alkaline...which promotes healthy cells.

In 1931 Dr. Otto Warburg won the Nobel Prize for discovering the cause of cancer: weakened cell respiration due to lack of oxygen on the cellular level -- this causes fermentation, which results in acidity, or low pH.

There is a close connection between the foods you eat and your pH balance. For example, Parmesan cheese is highly acid forming, -34; while spinach is an amazingly alkalizing food, +14.

When you get plenty of greens on a daily basis, you're able to better maintain a good alkaline pH balance.

5. Greens are made of chlorophyll...liquid sun energy.

As amazing as it may seem, the molecule of chlorophyll is strikingly similar to the molecule of human blood. Chlorophyll heals and cleanses your organs while destroying harmful substances.

Here are just a few of the powers of chlorophyll:

* Chlorophyll builds a high blood count

* Chlorophyll helps prevent cancer

* Chlorophyll counteracts toxins

* Chlorophyll promotes an alkaline body

* Chlorophyll helps sores heal faster

* Chlorophyll improves varicose veins

* Chlorophyll improves vision

Introducing The Green Smoothie: While the evidence for eating lots of greens continues to mount, who really wants to chomp through a pile of spinach everyday?

The solution is as convenient as it is efficient: *the green smoothie.*

Victoria discovered that when she blended greens with fruit and water, the result was an easily absorbed, delicious smoothie.

The key to reaping all the benefits from your green smoothies is to use a wide variety of greens and to drink it every day. Most enjoy it as a quick, nutrient-packed breakfast. *See the recipe in Chapter 10*

Victoria did a study where people drank green smoothies everyday for a month.

Most participants reported a noticeable increase in their energy levels after just the first week. This boost of energy may be just what you need to get into gear with your workouts.

Green Weight Loss

Need more convincing that greens should be a regular part of your diet?

People who consume green smoothies report fewer cravings for unhealthy food and tend to snack far less than when they aren't getting their greens.

So sip your green smoothie with a big smile knowing that you're turbo charging your health and expediting your weight loss.

How Healthy Is Your Salad?

Did you ever think that a salad could have more calories and fat than a serving of fried chicken?

Most people believe they're making a smart diet choice by opting for a salad but end up sabotaging their weight loss goals.

Don't get me wrong—salads are a great way to get your recommended daily allowance of fruits and veggies and are often full of nutritious goodness. Made with the right foods they can also be a great meal for those seeking to lose some weight.

Next time you inspect the salad bar or your refrigerator for ingredients to toss in your salad, keep the following tips in mind.

Fruits and Vegetables

Leafy greens and veggies should be the base of your salad. Choose as many vegetables as you would like. Choose from mixed greens, broccoli, sugar snap peas, spinach, cucumbers, onions, peppers, cauliflower, mushrooms, green beans, zucchini, shredded carrots, radish, sprouts, cabbage, beets, tomatoes, and whatever veggie you can think to add. At only 25 calories per serving, vegetables are loaded with vitamin C, folic acid, potassium, fiber, and antioxidants. So the more veggies, the better!

In addition to all your other veggies, go with the darkest green lettuce you can find. Choose Romaine, spinach, mustard leaves, or green leaf over iceberg for increased nutrition. Leafy greens come in at less than 20 calories per two cup serving and provide folic acid, antioxidants, vitamins, and minerals.

Fruit is also a great salad option, as they add sweetness and nutrition to your salad. Try fruit such as cranberries, grapes, sliced strawberries, tangerines, or apples, and watch your plain old salad transform into a piece of culinary art.

Protein

If you find yourself feeling hungry soon after eating a salad, add some protein the next time. Good sources of protein to toss in a healthy salad include hard-boiled eggs or just the egg whites, grilled chicken, grilled salmon, steamed or boiled shrimp, tuna packed in water, low-fat cottage cheese, or roasted turkey breast. A good serving size of this protein would be three ounces.

If meat or animal products aren't your thing, add about three quarters cup of one or more of these protein sources to your salad: lentils, tofu, black beans, garbanzo beans, chickpeas, or a small amount of nuts (they're also high in fat, so don't over-do.

Tempting as they may be, avoid fried, crispy, or saucy items that many add to salads (like croutons and bacon bits).

Extras

Though many salad extras may be packed with nutrition, they are often also full of calories. On average, extras add approximately 600 calories to an otherwise low-fat salad. A good rule of thumb when it comes to preparing a light salad is to choose just one high-calorie extra or two half-portion extras. Popular high-calorie add-ons include fried noodles, cottage cheese, pepperoni, avocado, bacon, blue cheese, croutons, cheese, or nuts.

If you love the taste and texture of croutons, try crushing a few and sprinkling them over your salad. If your salad doesn't seem complete without cheese, try a strong flavored cheese like Feta or Parmesan. A small amount will go far. Also, use chopped nuts instead of whole to get more bites of a good thing.

Dressing

Dressing often makes the salad. Unfortunately, it can also make a salad a high-calorie event. The average vinaigrette contains 50 calories in one tablespoon, while the same amount of ranch dressing contains about 90 calories. Plastic containers or dressing packets at restaurants contain four tablespoons of dressing. If you use the entire packet, you could add an additional 200-

360 calories. As if that weren't enough, many dressings also contain saturated fat. This raises cholesterol and the risk of heart disease.

Instead of grabbing the first dressing you see, look for a low-fat, low-calorie option. A healthy dressing choice is a couple teaspoons of olive oil mixed with vinegar or lemon and spices or herbs. Instead of drenching your salad in dressing, dip your fork into dressing before taking a bite of salad. Always have dressing on the side and never mixed in the salad.

Skinny Salad Dressing

Most of the fat and calories in salads are found in the dressing. Mix the following ingredients together for a guilt-free and delicious salad dressing:

1 cup fat free Greek Yogurt

3 Tablespoons white rice vinegar

1 shallot, minced

2 Packets Stevia

1 teaspoon oregano

1/2 teaspoon basil

1 clove garlic pressed

1 tsp sea salt

A dash of ground black pepper

Unleash the Power of Fiber

For most people, reckless snacking derails their healthy diet leaving them frustrated and overweight.

Do you eat a healthy lunch only to succumb to the vending machine an hour later?

I've got good news for you, if you do.

With just a few adjustments to your diet you can effortlessly kick your snacking habit to the curb.

You see, the urge to snack happens when your blood sugar levels drop—giving your body the message that you need more fuel. (Enter the vending machine.) This happens after eating meals that are low in fiber, low in calories, and high in sugar.

The solution?

Eat meals that are filled with fiber and you'll stabilize your blood sugar levels and feel full

---

longer.

The Case for High Fiber

Researchers have done their homework on fiber and the results spell easy weight loss for all who listen. By consuming an extra 14 grams of fiber each day you can cut your calorie intake by a full 10 percent.

People who consume more fiber (as low as 20 grams per day) weigh an average of eight pounds lighter than people who consume low fiber (closer to 10 grams per day).

There are two main reasons that high fiber leads to weight loss:

Fiber fills you up and stabilizes blood sugar for hours. This tames your appetite and protects you from needless snacking.

Foods that are high in fiber aren't as calorie dense. When you fill up on high fiber foods you eat just as much but take in fewer calories.

Breaking it Down

It's always easier to understand a concept like this when real life examples are given. So here's a review of a low fiber, high sugar diet that 'Jane' was eating, and then we'll see the small changes made to increase her fiber content and stabilize blood sugar.

Breakfast: Jane would typically eat a packet of instant oatmeal made with low fat milk and topped with banana and brown sugar. On the way to work she would also grab a mocha or latte.

Snack: Without fail by 10AM Jane's stomach would growl, sending her to the vending machine. She would end up with a small bag of chips, crackers, or candy to hold her over until lunch.

Lunch: By noon Jane was starving again and would inhale her packed lunch of a medium sized bagel with low fat cream cheese and deli slices and a small container of yogurt.

Snack: At 3PM, Jane's appetite would soar and she would scavenge the office for a small snack to hold her over until dinner. She usually found part of a leftover pastry or cookies and if all else failed she would once again turn to the vending machine.

Dinner: Most nights Jane would make a dinner of chicken breast, instant rice, and a small salad. Some nights she would substitute pasta for the rice.

Snack: Every night at 10PM Jane would find herself back in the kitchen in search of something sweet. Most often she would have a bowl of low fat ice cream or sorbet before going to bed.

Did you notice a trend in Jane's diet? While she kept her selections fairly low in fat, she hardly ate any fiber, which left her battling hunger all day. Her meals were also very high in sugar, which caused her blood sugar levels to jump up and plunge down throughout the day.

Here's the revised version of Jane's meals:

Breakfast: Instead of the instant oatmeal Jane switched to using old fashion (intact) oats. She then topped it with broken walnut pieces and banana. Instead of drinking a high-sugar mocha or latte, she started drinking hot tea.

Snack: Much to her surprise, 10PM came and went without so much as a hunger pain. Jane kept her focus and worked through till lunch.

Lunch: For lunch Jane had a cup of lentil soup, a slice of rye bread, and a cup of steamed veggies.

Snack: 3PM came and went and again Jane didn't feel the need snack. On her way home she ate a small handful of almonds.

Dinner: This meal didn't change much for Jane. Instead of instant rice she made brown or wild rice, and instead of white pasta she made whole wheat. She also added a vegetable dish to dinner in addition to the salad.

Snack: Most nights Jane skips her late night snack since she just doesn't feel hungry. On nights that she does want a sweet treat she enjoys sliced fruit.

That didn't look hard, did it?

As you probably noticed, Jane's daily calories dropped dramatically after adding fiber to each meal. Also her percentage of calories from fat also dropped since her snack foods were high in fat.

This means that Jane is effortlessly losing weight simply by consuming more fiber.

You can follow Jane's lead by evolving your diet to include higher levels of fiber.

Guilt Free Flavor

Looking to add flavor to your meal without adding extra calories? Try fresh herbs and spices. You will enjoy more flavor AND a smaller you! Remember to avoid creamy or oily dressings—while these are flavorful, they are also filled with fat and calories.

Veggie Power

According to WebMD, people who eat more fruits and vegetables as part of an overall healthy diet are likely to have a reduced risk of some chronic diseases.

Vegetables provide nutrients vital for maintaining a healthy body. Here are four quick tips for getting eating more vegetables:

Buy fresh vegetables in season. They cost less and taste better.

Buy vegetables that are quick to prepare. Pick up pre-washed bags of salad greens and add baby carrots and grape tomatoes for a simple salad.

Stock up on frozen vegetables for quick and easy cooking in the microwave.

Check out Chapter 10 for lots of veggie-filled recipes.

Lighten Up

Want to quickly eliminate fattening calories from your diet?

It's easy: simply don't add fat while cooking.

Instead of oils, butter, or lard, try cooking with a light cooking spray. Instead of frying, try broiling. Also drain or blot excess oil from food before eating it.

So that sums up what you should be eating, now let's discover what you should NEVER eat…

CHAPTER FOUR

Step # 3 - Why You Should Never, Ever Eat These Foods - EVER

After reading the previous section of what to eat, by process of elimination you've probably figured out what not to eat - -but let's still break it down.

Food manufactures have gotten so sneaky with their labels that you could eat a snack comprised of processed grains and corn syrup with artificial flavors and think that you just ate something healthy.

Then, as your weight crept up, you'd wonder why.

Read on to discover which foods to never eat...

Never Eat These 5 Foods

The world of fitness and weight loss is often confusing, with contradictory information swirling about. I'm going to cut through the confusion and make things really simple for you.

Below is a list of five foods that you should never eat.

These foods will derail your fitness and weight loss efforts every single time.

In addition, I will suggest a healthy substitute for each of these off-limit foods.

By simply swapping out the items below you will quickly and effortlessly become healthier, leaner and fitter than you are today.

Do-Not-Eat #1: Anything Fried

Fried food is loaded with fat and calories while offering zero nutritional value. It's a lose-lose! Sure, fries and chips TASTE good, but healthier items also taste good. Just say no to the deep fried items on your menu. You'll be thinner and healthier and as a bonus won't have greasy fingers.

Try This #1: Broiled

If you simply must have a French fry, then make them at home in your oven. Use sweet potatoes as these are a more complex carbohydrate. Cut into matchsticks, drizzle with a tablespoon of olive oil along with a dash of salt, then place in your oven on broil. Mix every 5 minutes until the fries are tender on the inside and crispy on the outside.

Do-Not-Eat #2: White Bread

White bread products have zero nutritional value and are quickly converted by your body into sugar. So you may as well eat a cupcake. Even breads that are technically wheat, but are as soft and smooth as white bread, should be avoided. Don't be afraid to discard the bread from your sandwich or to push away that bread basket. Your waist will shrink and you'll lose that bloated feeling that high carbohydrate meals give you.

Try This #2: Sprouted Grain Bread

If you must have bread, then stick with sprouted. Sprouted grain bread is a lot easier on your digestion and is packed full of nutrients. Two delicious brands are Food For Life's Ezekiel bread and Manna Organics. Sprouted grain breads are often kept in the freezer section since they don't contain preservatives to prolong shelf life.

Do-Not-Eat #3: Creamy Salad Dressing

You were so good to order a salad, but then you ruined it by drenching the salad in fattening creamy dressing. Just a few tablespoons of creamy dressing contain more than 20 grams of fat and hundreds of calories.

Try This #3: Vinegar Dressing

Salad dressing is meant to lend flavor to the salad, not fat and calories. Vinegar-based dressings pack amazing flavor with minimal fat and calories. You can even mix your own dressing at home. Take high quality vinegar, fresh lemon juice, salt and pepper, your choice of dried herbs, and a bit of olive oil.

Do-Not-Eat #4: White Rice

I'm sure by now you've heard that white rice is not a healthy choice. Just like white bread, white rice has zero nutritional value – other than calories. Fiber and vitamins have been removed and the glycemic load will quickly prime your body for storing fat.

Try This #4: Brown Rice

Brown rice has three times the amount of fiber, more B vitamins as well as other nutrients, won't sky rocket your blood, and will keep you feeling fuller longer. That should be enough to convince you to swap your large pile of white rice out for a small pile of brown rice.

Do-Not-Eat #5: White Sugar

Sugar and high fructose corn syrup are the epitome of anti-fitness food. Nothing will destroy your progress, expand your waist and plummet your energy levels like sugar will. If you only take away one do-not-eat food from this article please let it be sugar.

Try This #5: Fruit

Don't turn to artificial sweeteners to get your sweet fix. Instead, turn to nature's wholesome source of sugar, fruit. Eat organic fruit that is seasonal and locally grown. Stay away from dried fruit and fruit juices, as these are high in simple calories.

4 Worst Breakfast Items

Don't get caught eating one of these 4 things for breakfast:

Breakfast pastry: muffins, donuts, bear claws, and croissants sure taste good with coffee, but all those refined carbs are going to cause unwanted weight gain.

Granola Bars: watch out for the breakfast bars that claim to give you fiber, vitamins and minerals. Check the number of carbs and sugars on the back of the label – most contain the same sugar as a pastry.

Cereal: here's another popular breakfast item that has tons of sugar lurking beneath its surface. Only eat cereal that has no added sugar and contains some protein and healthy fat.

Drive Thru Breakfast Sandwich: don't even think about heading to the drive thru for a quick breakfast sandwich. Instead, grab a hard-boiled egg or Greek yogurt from home to enjoy on your commute.

This One's For Your Sweet Tooth

Your sweet tooth has gotten you into lots of trouble over the years.

Think about all those diets you abandoned for a slice of cake and all the extra calories you took in 'just to have a taste of something sweet' before bed.

Where has it gotten you?

Into pants that are another size larger. Into your doctor's office for another lecture. Into a body that you no longer enjoy.

Yes, sweet treats sure are tempting, but the life-long repercussions far outweigh the momentary pleasure.

To help you conquer your sweet tooth, I've identified the five sweet traps you should avoid, as well as a healthy substitute for each.

Sweet Trap #1: Candy

Nothing gets refined sugar circulating through your body quicker than a fistful of candy and if you're in the habit of eating candy daily then your body will crave it.

Candy has virtually no nutritional value, other than caloric energy, and will quickly end up stored on your body in the form of unwanted, annoying fat.

Try This: Swap your sickly-sweet candy out for a handful of unsalted nuts, a few pieces of unsweetened, dried fruit, or a small square of very dark chocolate (at least 72% cocoa content).

Sweet Trap #2: Baked Goods

Cake, cookies, brownies, pastries, donuts, and pies are popular vehicles for sugar consumption. While these may not taste as sweet as candy, the combination of refined sugar and white flour will spike your blood sugar just the same.

Very much like candy, regularly eating baked goods may become a habit. Break yourself of this and you'll find the number on your scale going down rather than up.

Try This: Put down the cookie and reach for a piece of fresh, seasonal fruit. Fruit is nature's candy and is every bit as blissful as a slice of cake. Serving a beautiful fruit platter to guests can be as delightful as any baked treat.

Sweet Trap #3: Ice Cream

Nothing makes you feel as happy and carefree as a bowl of creamy ice cream…until that ice cream makes its permanent home on your waist. Very much like candy, ice cream has few nutritional benefits.

Try This: Let's face it, cold, creamy, and sweet makes a delicious combination. Create a healthy protein-packed ice cream with the recipe on page 237.

Sweet Trap #4: Soda Pop

A regular can of soda pop contains the equivalent of 10 packets of sugar. That's more sugar than you should consume in a week's time!

Soda pop is something that you get into the habit of drinking and so without thinking. The good news is that a habit can be broken and then replaced with something healthier.

Try This: Take soda pop out of your diet. Period. There are plenty of other, healthier, beverages available to you. Try the recipes for Spa Water below.

Sweet Trap #5: Blended Drinks

Smoothies, blended coffee drinks, and milkshakes are all tempting treats especially in hot summer months. Don't give in to the temptation!

These items are even more deadly than most treats since they are consumed through a straw and don't make you feel full. Let me assure you that even though you don't feel full, like you would after a piece of cake, you're still taking in a boatload of sugary calories.

Try This: Make your own healthy blended drinks at home by using natural sweeteners like stevia or simply by using fruit. Take the ice cream recipe below, add non-fat milk and mix in the blender for a high protein milkshake.

Eliminating refined sugar from your diet will do so much for your health as well as your weight.

A great thing to remember is that once you've fallen out of the habit of eating sugar, your body will no longer crave it.

This means that each day spent in discipline will bring you closer to the day that sugar no longer has a hold over you. Imagine how much slimmer and healthier you will be!

Beyond Soda

You know that soda pop isn't good for you…and yet you still drink it.

I understand that plain water gets boring – especially when you're having a party or gathering.

Use the recipes for "Spa Water" below and quickly turn plain water into an exciting and refreshing treat without added sugar or chemicals:

Citrus: Slice an orange, lemon, and lime into a large pitcher of water. Add ice; allow to chill for 1 hour before serving.

Raspberry Lime: Slice a lime into a large pitcher of water, add a handful of raspberries. Add ice; allow to chill for 1 hour before serving.

Strawberry Basil: Slice 10 strawberries into a large pitcher of water, add 5 leaves of basil. Add ice; allow to chill for 1 hour before serving.

Watermelon Rosemary: Place ½ cup of small watermelon chunks into a large pitcher of water, add two sprigs of rosemary. Add ice and allow to chill for 1 hour before serving.

Pineapple Mint: Place ½ cup of small pineapple chunks into a large pitcher of water, add 15 mint leaves. Add ice and allow to chill for 1 hour before serving.

What You Don't Know Could Hurt You

How much thought do you put into what you eat?

If you want to get into great shape then you'll be interested to know that 80% of your fitness results are attributed to your diet.

In our fast-paced society, eating is often done with little or no thought as to what exactly it is being ingested. Excess body fat is a direct outcome of this hurried, poor nutrition. Even if you have the best intentions with your diet, you are likely frustrated and fed up with extra pounds.

I don't blame you for being confused about what you should eat. The media surely doesn't help. One day the talking heads want you to give up all fats. The next day carbs are the culprit and then acai berries become the holy grail of weight loss.

The food manufacturers increase confusion by printing misleading labels and bogus health claims.

Sometimes it seems like the whole system is set up to confuse and frustrate us into buying the latest and greatest packaged food.

The bottom line is that your physique is largely a result of what you eat, so the foods that you put into your body should be carefully selected.

It's time to re-examine what you eat.

It all starts with reading nutritional labels. The nutritional content and ingredient list will give you everything you need to know about the quality of the food item.

I've outlined 5 ingredients that should raise a red flag when you turn over that package and find them listed:

Red Flagged Ingredient #1: High Fructose Corn Syrup (HFCS)

HFCS is a manmade sugar derived predominantly from genetically modified corn. The sweet concoction has been shown to promote binges and hysterical hunger and wreaks havoc on your blood sugar levels, promoting fat storage.

The introduction of HFCS into our food supply directly paralleled a 47% spike in Type 2 Diabetes cases as well as an 80% increase in obesity.

Food manufacturers use HFCS in many mainstream products, including the following:

- Sauces (including ketchup)
- Yogurt
- Energy Bars
- Soft Drinks / Fruit Juices
- Processed baked goods
- Cereals
- Crackers

- Ice Cream
- Salad Dressing
- Most packaged snack foods

Red Flagged Ingredient #2: Hydrogenated Fat / Partially Hydrogenated Fat (Trans Fat)

Hydrogenated and partially hydrogenated fats have undergone such extensive processing that the chemical structure has changed from a "cis" shape, which the human body recognizes and utilizes, to a "trans" shape, which is foreign and destructive to human physiology.

Check each food label for the word 'hydrogenated' and avoid it diligently. Cutting out hydrogenated fats is a simple step towards looking and feeling your best.

Red Flagged Ingredient #3: Aspartame

Aspartame is an artificial sweetener that was denied eight times by the FDA before being approved in 1973. Many scientists objected the approval claiming that aspartame hadn't been proven safe for use as a food additive.

MIT neuroscientist, Richard Wurtman, researched the effects of aspartame and concluded that it promotes cravings for foods high in calories and carbohydrates.

Though aspartame is calorie-free it still causes insulin to be released, which its job is to stow away sugar – when this sugar is not available, the result is often hypoglycemia and severe hunger. Not exactly a recipe for weight loss.

Red Flagged Ingredient #4: White Sugar

White sugar comes from the juice of a sugar cane plant that has undergone an intensive refining process. In this process all of the enzymes, fiber, vitamins, and minerals are destroyed, rendering it nutritionally void.

White sugar is also extremely high in calories, which your body loves to store away in fat cells.

Refined sugar has been linked to a weakened immune system, hyperactivity, ADD, mental and emotional disorders, dental cavities, hypoglycemia, enlargement of the liver and kidneys, and an imbalance of neurotransmitters in the brain. All that and it leads to weight gain.

Red Flagged Ingredient #5: White Flour

White flour comes from natural whole wheat that has been stripped of nutrients, vitamins and minerals. This results in a nutritionally void product that is packed with calories that release quickly into your system, creating a spike in blood sugar. As you know, this promotes fat storage and leads to hysterical hunger and cravings. You don't need that.

Once you cut these five items out of your diet, you'll be pleased with the results. Expect to lose weight, to have more energy, and to feel better than you have in a long time.

If you're serious about looking and feeling your best through purifying your diet, then focus on eating real food items. Real foods include lean meats, vegetables, whole grains, fruits, nuts, and seeds.

Are These 3 Foods Making You Fat?

It's easy to let yourself be fooled into thinking the things you eat are healthy. Foods dressed in crafty packaging lead you to believe they will help you lose weight.

But do they?

The truth is that most of the time the only thing special about the so-called healthy food product is the clever marketing. Have you been fooled by the following foods?

So-Called Healthy Food #1: SALAD

Who doesn't get a self-righteous feeling when ordering a salad, right? Salads are healthy, and salads equal weight loss. Unfortunately, not anymore.

Salad in and of itself is a wonderful, healthy food. It is filled with nutrients and untouched by artificial additives. If only we left it at that.

Most salads on the menu today are loaded with fat laden extras. Croutons, tortilla strips, nuts, and even fried chicken (not the best source of protein). And let's not forget the salad dressing.

While you know that salad dressing isn't very healthy, you may not be aware of the staggering number of fat calories packed in these dressings. Most people add between a quarter to a half a cup of dressing to their salad, and with the average creamy salad dressing weighing in at 8-12 grams of fat per tablespoon, you can see how an innocent collection of greens can quickly turn into a spare tire.

So-Called Healthy Food #2: 100 CALORIE PACKS

In the snack section of your local grocery store you've probably seen the attractively packaged "100 Calorie Packs." These light and airy snack packs send a subtle message that they are healthy and in line with your desire to drop the fat. I mean, how harmful can they be? Let's take a look at the snacks within the package.

Here are the most popular:

- Oreo cookies

- Ritz snack mix
- Planter's peanut butter cookies
- Cheese Nips crackers
- Chips Ahoy cookies
- Shortbread cookie

Hmmm, that list sounds like junk food—doesn't it? These items are high in sugar, salt, and fat, and they don't contain a grain of nutritional value. And let's be honest, most people don't eat just one pack…

So-Called Healthy Food #3: CEREAL

Can a box of cereal help you lose weight? That's the message being sent out by a handful of cereal brands, namely Special K. This cereal manufacturer has gone so far as to create the Special K Challenge, a program which claims to help drop 6 pounds in 2 weeks. The message that most consumers take away from the cereal commercials is "If I eat this brand of cereal then I will lose weight."

Wait! Don't grab a bowl of your favorite cereal along with your skinny jeans just yet.

It's dangerous to think that any food item will promote weight loss, especially a food item that is high in simple carbohydrates. In the fine print you will see that the cereal claims to help lose weight when incorporated with a very low calorie diet and that the cereal itself has no weight loss inducing power.

Not Too Sweet

If want to lose weight, cut the sugar out of your diet. Sugar encourages fat storage by causing your insulin levels to rise. Try natural low-calorie alternatives to sugar, such as stevia.

The Liquid Calorie Ban

Here's an easy way to live healthier: don't drink calories.

Liquid calories are sneaky.

You don't get that full feeling like with solid foods, but you're still taking in tons of calories.

Avoid drinks like: regular sodas, smoothies, juices, sweet coffee drinks, hot chocolate, milk shakes, and alcoholic beverages. Drink plenty of water instead—you'll lose weight and feel great.

The Sweetest Scam of All Time

The correct answer to the following question will shock you.

Would you survive longer on a diet of just water OR on a diet of water and refined sugar?

The answer: You would survive longer on just water.

Sound impossible? Just ask the five sailors who were shipwrecked in 1793.

The ship was filled with sugar, thus giving the marooned five a diet of sugar and water. When they were finally picked up, nine days later, they were in a wasted condition due to starvation.

The story of the five sailors intrigued French physiologist Francois Magendie to conduct a series of experiments in which he fed dogs a diet of sugar. All of the dogs died.

Magendie proved that as a steady diet, refined sugar is worse than nothing.

How can sugar be worse than nothing? Plainly put, refined sugar is an anti-nutrient.

It starts out as sugar cane and then goes through an extensive refining process that destroys all of the enzymes, fiber, vitamins, and minerals. What you're left with are empty, naked calories.

The problem is that your body needs the enzymes, fiber, vitamins and minerals that were taken out in the refining process in order to metabolize sugar and use it as energy, so it takes those nutrients from your own body.

So, while you are enjoying that chocolate bar, sugar is draining vital nutrients from your body, like a sweet parasite.

And it doesn't end there…

Sugar creates false hunger (as a result of the insulin rush and then ensuing plummet in your blood sugar levels), which makes you overeat. This means a constant struggle with your weight in which you never seem to achieve your ideal size.

Sugar promotes aging (due to the advanced glycation end products, or AGEs, that occur when insulin levels are consistently elevated as a result of eating too much sugar). Sugar has even been dubbed the negative fountain of youth.

Sugar weakens your bones –making you vulnerable for osteoporosis and weakens your teeth—making you vulnerable for cavities (both due to the calcium being pulled from your bones and teeth in order for your body to process sugar).

Sugar in excess is stored as fat (after your liver has no more room to store it, sugar is converted to fat and deposited on your belly, thighs, hips, and the backs of your arms).

Sugar can impair brain functioning (as a result of depleted B-vitamin production).

If you're still not convinced of the danger of sugar, here are more ailments linked to its overconsumption: varicose veins, constipation, hormonal imbalances, ADD and ADHD, increased emotional instability, depressed immune system, increased risk of cancer and degenerative diseases.

The average modern person consumes 46 teaspoons of sugar every day. That comes out to roughly 175 pounds of sugar each year.

And it's no wonder since the sugar industry is big business. They sneak sugar into any product that they can.

Go through the foods in your home and you'll see that sugar has been added to everything from ketchup and spaghetti sauce to crackers, oatmeal, peanut butter and even 'healthy' items like weight loss bars.

Where does this leave you?

You are in a unique position. Your personal judgment determines the foods that you eat and the foods that you avoid. It is my hope that you approach sugar with new eyes.

While all other foods offer you caloric energy PLUS some nutritional benefit, sugar DOES NOT. Sugar is simply caloric energy with a sweet habit forming taste and a hoard of health risks.

Use your judgment wisely and limit your sugar consumption – you'll love the benefits of low sugar living.

(Oh and if you're ever in a shipwreck with only sugar and water at your disposal – just drink the water!)

The Many Names of Sugar

While you're checking out nutrition labels for sugar content be on the lookout for the following names that all describe refined sugar:

- Sucrose
- High fructose corn syrup
- Fructose
- Lactose
- Organic sugar
- Maltose
- Dextrose
- Glucose

The Deep Fried Disaster

I am often asked how to lose weight quickly and easily.

Of course no one wants to listen to a lecture on the importance of healthy eating coupled with a solid exercise routine. That would preclude the quick and easy part.

So in a world where two thirds of all adults are overweight or obese, and some doctors predict that we will soon see a generation with a lower life expectancy than their parents due to obesity related diseases, I've come up with a solution that is both quick and easy. (Drum roll, please.)

Stop eating fried foods. (Gasp!)

Fried foods, despite having little to no nutritional value and being loaded with fat and calories, have become an accepted indulgence in our society. It's so accepted that many restaurants serve fries or chips alongside every meal.

It's no wonder that fried foods are the number one thing that most people crave – they are salty, addictive, and plentiful.

Are Fried Foods Really That Bad?

In a nutshell, yes; fried foods really are that bad for you.

Take an average potato, bake it and you have 110 calories and 0 grams of fat. Take that same potato, turn it into French fries and you have 380 calories and 18 grams of fat.

Frying food is the easiest way to dramatically increase the calorie and fat content. And you know that extra calories and fat end up as extra body fat.

Other disasters that fried foods put you at risk for include:

- Heart Disease

- Diabetes

- Clogged Arteries

- High Blood Pressure

- Obesity

- Acne

- Fried foods have also been known to trigger Acid Reflux and IBS (Irritable Bowel Syndrome).

Need I say more?

Going Fried-Free

Giving up fried food may not be easy, though it will arguably be one of the best things you do for your health and appearance. You *will* lose weight and improve your health by eliminating fried food from your life.

Keep in mind that, like all habits, the first 30 days will be the toughest. Make things easier by staying away from situations that place you in front of a big basket of fries or plate of donuts.

New Foods to Love

Instead of fried foods, enjoy the following:

Substitute a salad or fruit instead of fries

Baked potato – but pass on the butter and sour cream

Baked chicken instead of fried chicken

Baked chips instead of fried chips

Raw veggie pieces

You may be surprised how delicious these healthier options taste.

Help, I'm addicted!

If your diet has consistently included fried foods—multiple times a day or several times each week, then giving it up may take more work than simply trying healthier options.

You'll need to use some mental strategies as well.

To do this focus on all the negative things about eating fried foods:

Think of how bloated and heavy you feel afterward

Remember the heart burn you've experienced

Focus on the extra pounds you want to lose – imagine donuts and French fries sticking to your belly and thighs

Look at your acne

Feel the discomfort of being out of breath doing normal activities

You didn't think I was really going to skip telling you how beneficial exercise is to achieving your health and weight loss goals did you?

The bottom line is that exercise plus healthy eating will give you the body that you want.

What are you waiting for? Drop that bag of chips and change your life!

The Trans-Fat-Free Decoy

You've probably heard that many restaurants and food manufacturers have stopped using trans-fats.

Don't get too excited.

While trans fats aren't as bad as other fats, fried items are is still loaded with fat, calories, and sodium – all things that you want to avoid when trying to lose weight.

Before you eat a trans-fat-free item check the overall nutritional content.

Does it contain saturated fat? What is the total fat and calorie count? What about sugar and sodium?

Don't let a trans-fat-free label distract you from the overall nutritional content of the food.

#1 Rule Of Clean Eating: No Refined Sugar

I can't say enough about the dangers of refined sugar.

Regular sugar consumption will always cause weight gain. In addition to ruining your figure, chronic sugar consumption puts you at risk of numerous health problems.

When you're in the habit of taking in sugar everyday it's hard to quit, but once you've broken the habit you won't give sugar a second thought.

Whenever your sweet tooth flares up eat a piece of fresh organic fruit.

Let's move on and discuss when and how much you should be eating…

CHAPTER FIVE

Step #4 - Figuring Out When and How Much to Eat to Lose Maximum Fat

Here's the part of most diet plans where it gets really complicated and confusing.

I've got awesome news for you about the *Fit Body Boot Camp Unstoppable Fat Loss Formula*.

When you follow the guidelines for what to eat and what not to eat, the when and how much of your diet plan doesn't matter too much. You'll begin to shed fat immediately once you switch the contents of your diet.

Let's get into the nitty-gritty of when and how much to eat....

When to eat

It's been said that your metabolism is like a campfire and that to maintain a consistent burn you should eat at regular intervals throughout the day.

This analogy works; however, rather than basing your snack and meal times by the clock, it's more effective to listen to your body's own signals of hunger.

How much to eat

By eating the right foods you will naturally begin to eat fewer calories.

Fiber-rich vegetables, which are a huge part of the *Unstoppable Fat Loss Formula* eating guide, are very low in calories.

Sugar-laden and processed foods, which you now avoid, are calorie-dense.

Your body thrives on the natural, whole foods described in Chapter 3 and since you no longer indulge in the foods discussed in Chapter 4 then natural fat loss will happen organically.

I'm not going to tell you exactly when and how much to eat, but I do want to discuss the obstacle of overeating.

Most people never make it to their goals because they get caught up in eating too many calories.

The good news is that by sticking with the foods outlined in Chapter 3 you'll be less likely to overindulge.

Here's what you need to know about overeating...

The Art of Eating Mindfully

Do you ever find yourself snacking away without paying attention to how much you're eating?

Maybe you're focused on a movie or a ball game. This is a sure-fire way to gain weight.

When your goal is to drop pounds it is important to practice the art of eating mindfully.

This means that when you eat you should stay tuned in to your level of satiety so that at the first sign of fullness you will stop.

The 7 Deadly Dieting Mistakes

It's a common problem. You've been on a diet for weeks and aren't losing weight like you thought you would.

It may be because you're consuming more calories than you think.

Keep reading to discover seven sneaky habits that may be sabotaging your weight loss efforts.

Mistake #1: Forgetting Liquid Calories

It's easy to forget that the things you drink have calories—some more than you'd think. In fact, some beverages have more calories than an entire plate of food.

It is estimated that around 20 percent of your daily calories come from what you drink. So as you drink your juice with breakfast, rehydrate with a sports drink at the gym, or drink a glass of wine at dinner, think about the calories you're adding.

For calories' sake, it's best to avoid all sweetened sodas, sweetened or flavored coffee drinks, sweetened tea, and smoothies. Replace these high-calorie drinks with water, skim milk, and unsweetened herbal tea. Because while they taste great, liquids generally don't satisfy hunger, so they are just empty calories.

Mistake #2 Meal Skipping

Many dieters think they'll cut their calorie intake by skipping a meal, usually breakfast.

But this is a big mistake.

Research has shown that those who skip breakfast actually weigh more than those who eat three meals a day. Skipping a meal usually causes you to eat more calories during the day because you will end up eating even more food later in the day because you're so hungry.

So aim to eat four to six meals a day including healthy snacks (see page for healthy snacks). A healthy breakfast that will keep you feeling full all morning contains protein and fiber. An example would be whole-wheat toast and an egg.

Mistake #3: Oversized Portions

Just because restaurants load your plate with a mountain of food doesn't mean you should eat that much at home for a normal meal.

Remember that your stomach, like your heart, is the size of your fist. Don't think you could fit much food into your fist? You're right. And contrary to what mama taught you as a child, you don't have to eat all the food in front of you.

To eat a little less, use smaller plates and eat slower so you know when you're full. The golden rule is to chew each bite 20 times. Also, remember that portion control applies to healthy foods as well, as they also contain calories.

Mistake #4: Too Many Extra

A salad is a healthy, low calorie option. At least until you add dressing, bacon, cheese, and croutons.

These add extra calories fast.

One tablespoon of dressing contains 75 to 100 calories. With that in mind, it's no wonder grilled-chicken salads at a fast-food restaurant can have more calories than a hamburger.

Mistake #5: Blaming Your Genes

Many people give up on dieting or think there's no hope when it comes to meeting their goal weight because of their genes.

Just like you may share your father's hair color or your mother's eye color, there is a small chance you also share your parent's body type. However, this is no excuse for not doing anything about trying to lose weight.

Stick to your diet and exercise plan and you should definitely see results.

Mistake #6: Eating Without Thinking

It happens to everyone. You're tired after a long day and you just want to veg in front of the television or read a good book. Unfortunately, mindlessly eating is often involved. You may think that since it's not on a plate it doesn't matter, but every bite you take counts.

When it comes to a successful diet, make rules for appropriate times to eat. And don't always feel the need to eat when relaxing. Try sipping on water or tea, chewing gum, or simply don't put anything in your mouth.

Mistake #7: Eliminating All Treats

Dieters often become overzealous in their plan and completely rid the house of all the food they enjoy, whether chips, sweets, snacks, or any high calorie food.

This commitment may last a few days until you can't tolerate it any longer and you overindulge on what you deprived yourself of.

A better plan is to allow yourself a treat every once in a while.

Remember that everyone makes mistakes, but be smart and don't let these common pitfalls keep your from meeting your weight loss goal!

The Top 5 Ways You Eat Too Much

Each day you make well over 200 decisions about food, according to Brian Wansink, PH.D. in his book, *Mindless Eating*. Your weight is the sum total of your past food decisions.

According to Wansink, overeating can be greatly reduced simply by removing the cues in your environment that cause you to overeat.

He goes on to explain the top 5 Diet Danger Zones and the solutions for each:

The Meal Stuffer: At mealtime you really stuff yourself. You clean everything off your plate, eat quickly and often go back for seconds. You consider yourself to have a "healthy appetite" and often feel uncomfortably full after eating.

Use the Half-Plate Rule: fill half of your plate with vegetables and the other half with protein and starch.

Use smaller plates and wait 20 minutes before deciding if you want seconds.

Eat slower so your appetite can catch up with what you've already eaten.

Don't place serving dishes on the table. Pre-plate your food and then put the rest out of reach.

The Snack Grazer: You eat whatever food is within reach and snack at least three times throughout the day. You can't walk past a candy dish without dipping in. Your snacking is rarely done out of hunger. Here are some tips to avoid snacking:

Chew gum throughout your day to avoid mindless munching.

Keep tempting snack foods out of sight and out of mind.

Never eat directly from a package. Portion out your snack into a dish.

Don't purchase tempting snack foods for future snacking. Keep a wide variety of fruits and vegetables on hand instead.

The Party Binger: Whenever you attend a social event where the main attraction is food, you eat without stopping. With all the distraction you quickly lose track of how much you've consumed and often stop only when it's time to leave.

Stay more than an arm's length away from the buffet or snack bowls.

Put only two food items on your plate during each trip to the table.

Make yourself feel full by eating the big healthy stuff first, like broccoli and carrots.

Remind yourself why you are at the party; first to socialize or to conduct business and secondarily to eat.

The Restaurant Indulger: You eat out at least three times a week and enjoy every minute of it. You love appetizers, large entrees, and rich desserts. When you leave the table you are always stuffed.

Ask your waiter to remove the bread basket from the table.

Before you eat, ask your waiter to box half of your entrée to take home.

Decide to either share an appetizer or a dessert, never have both.

Skip the appetizer menu and instead start your meal with a side salad.

The Desktop (or Dashboard) Diner: You like to multi-task by eating at your desk or on the go. Your lightning-quick meals are grabbed on-the-go from fast food joints, vending machines, and convenience stores. You don't plan your meals ahead of time and end up eating whatever you can quickly find.

Pack a healthy lunch and bring it with you.

Stock your work area with healthy protein-filled snacks.

Drink plenty of water throughout the day.

Turn off the computer or pull your car over while you eat.

By making these healthy changes when it comes to your food decisions, you will put yourself back on course and moving in the direction of healthy weight loss.

A Simple Mind Shift (The Secret Tid Bit)

Want to eat less without feeling deprived? This simple mind shift will help you do just that.

Instead of eating until you feel full, stop eating as soon as you are no longer hungry. Yes, there's a difference.

3 Steps to Overcome Overeating

Let's face it; the extra pounds you're carrying around are due to overeating – plain and simple.

Why do you overeat? Here are a few likely reasons:

Habit: Whether you realize it or not, you eat in a learned pattern rather than out of need. You clean your plate because that's what your mother taught you to do. You eat what is served without stopping to check if you are full. You butter two pieces of toast for breakfast rather than questioning if one piece would do the job.

Absentminded: You forget to pay attention when you eat. Mindless munching while watching a movie, snacking while driving, or picking at food while cooking – these absentminded calories really add up.

Something Deeper: Sometimes you use food for recreation or to change your mood. These calories may lend you a temporary sense of comfort or pleasure, but ultimately your body suffers from the indulgence.

Here are **3 Steps To Overcome Overeating** – read these, and apply them to your life.

Step #1: Pay Attention

Be aware of what and how much you eat. This simple concept will save you from hundreds upon hundreds of calories each week.

To apply this rule, don't eat while your attention is distracted by another activity. Only put food in your mouth when you are hungry and conscious of it. This means turn off the T.V., get out of your car, and no matter what you do, don't graze in the kitchen while cooking.

Step #2: Practice Balance

Be aware of the types of food that you eat during each meal and make sure that it's balanced. When you eat a balanced diet filled with lean protein, whole grains, lots of veggies, a few daily servings of fruit, and limited fat and sweets, your body will be satisfied and you'll lose the urge to overeat.

This means you shouldn't always eat carb-based meals nor should you always eat high-fat meals. Make a mental checklist of the food groups that you've eaten each day. Did you eat lean protein? Did you have plenty of vegetables? Did you refrain from eating more than one or two primarily carb-based meals? This mental checklist will save you from making food decisions that you'd later regret.

Step #3: Be Tuned In

Your body will always tell you when its hunger has been satisfied – you've just gotten so good at ignoring the signs that you barrel through your meal only to feel like you've been hit by a ton of bricks once all that food hits your stomach. It's time to take a deep breath and listen to your body.

An important part of being tuned in is to eat slowly. Once you start to pay attention you'll notice a point when each bite becomes less and less satisfying. That is your body's way of letting you know that you've had enough and that each continued bite is simply overkill (yes, even if you're only halfway through that plate of pasta).

By learning how to control your eating habits, you'll find weight loss to come simply and naturally.

No More Clean Plates

You know that portions are now larger than ever. Do you really need to eat all of that food?

Of course you don't.

It is time to release yourself from the obligation to eat every morsel on your plate. Start by always leaving one or two bites. Soon you will find that you naturally stop eating when you're full – even if your plate isn't empty.

The Last Weight Loss Tip You'll Ever Need

By now you've just about had it.

You've been exercising and eating healthy for ages, but haven't met your weight loss goal.

What gives?

It's an issue that every whole-grain-veggie-and-lean-meat-eating health-seeker faces at some point in their fitness journey.

Until you come face-to-face with one ugly truth about yourself, you'll always be stuck in this limbo of doing the right thing, eating healthy and yet not having the stunning body to show for it.

Once you conquer this last issue, you'll quickly achieve your ultimate goal and will slide into the on-going maintenance phase.

Here's your problem: You eat too many calories.

That's it.

Master this problem and you'll quickly and easily achieve the body of your dreams.

"But I only eat healthy calories, so quantity doesn't really matter," you're thinking.

While I applaud you for eating healthy calories, you're fooling yourself if you think quantity isn't an issue.

Calorie Counting Works

Have you heard of the professor from Kansas State University, Mark Haub, and his famous junk food diet?

As an experiment for his nutrition class, Haub put himself on a diet of almost exclusively candy bars, packaged cakes, and processed snacks. The catch was that he only ate 1800 calories each day. His previous diet of normal and healthy foods was about 2600 calories each day.

Within two months Haub had lost 30 pounds and his BMI dropped from the overweight category down to normal.

While I would never recommend eating junk food, this is quite a dramatic demonstration of how reduced calorie intake works for weight loss.

How many calories do you eat each day?

If you don't know the answer, then get excited because this one weight loss tool will change everything for you.

Start Your Food Journal

Food journaling used to be a cumbersome act that involved lugging around a journal, writing down each food item throughout the day and then looking everything up at the end of the day to manually tally calories.

Not so anymore.

Today food journaling has gone digital. Tracking calories takes only seconds of your time.

Download a food journal application to your smart phone and at the touch of your fingers you'll be able to look up food items and instantly see your running calorie tally.

Meet with your doctor to determine a daily calorie count that will allow for safe weight loss and diligently maintain that number. Eat healthy, fresh foods and when you decide to indulge, do so within your target calorie range.

This one small, proactive step will give you structure and clarity when it comes to making food choices and will quickly result in pounds lost and goals achieved.

Once your goal weight is met, your target calorie range will be adjusted for maintenance.

5 Steps to Curb Closet Eating

Do the following statements describe you?

I prefer to eat in private where no one else can see.

I eat healthy in front of others but then indulge recklessly in private.

I follow a healthy diet during the day, only to fall off the wagon at night.

I sneak food secretly and eat it away from others.

If you can relate to any of the above statements then you may be engaging in closet eating. This "secret eating life" of yours sabotages your fitness goals, making it impossible to achieve the body that you want.

Before we dive into this topic, it's important to approach yourself from a place of love and respect. Resist the urge to look at yourself as a failure as you strive to discard unhealthy eating habits.

Use the following 5 steps to curb your closet eating once and for all:

Step #1: Learn Your Triggers

Journal about the feelings you experience before, during, and after an episode of closet eating. Was there a particular trigger that caused you to feel stressed, or angry, or helpless before the urge to eat in secrecy hit you?

Refer back to your journal after a handful of episodes and try to determine a pattern. This will allow you to prepare yourself with an exit plan before the next potential episode.

For example, if you find that your closet eating occurs mainly when your spouse goes out of town on business, then make plans to visit with friends rather than be alone at home with food.

Step #2: Log Every Calorie

Let's face the facts. Just because no one sees you eat it, doesn't mean that the calories don't exist. The simple act of tallying each food item that you eat will force you to be more mindful of your eating habits.

Find your ideal calorie range by consulting your doctor and be aware of how close you come to that range each day. Resist the urge to not log foods that are eaten in secrecy.

The point is to bring accountability to the situation, so be vigilant.

Step #3: Carry Healthy Snacks

When the urge to eat in secrecy hits you, it may be useful to allow yourself the snack, but change the script slightly by making it healthy and portion controlled (see snack list below).

Eat one of these snacks every few hours to prevent from becoming overly hungry, thus more susceptible to reckless eating.

Enjoy your healthy snack very slowly, then wait 20 minutes before deciding if you are full or still hungry.

A small handful of raw almonds

1 small apple with a tablespoon of peanut butter

¼ cup of hummus and a few carrot sticks

5 olives

1 cup unshelled edamame

2 ounces of sliced turkey breast

1 cup plain Greek yogurt and ¼ cup berries

Step #4: Don't Stock Bad Food

Most cases of closet eating are said to occur in the comfort of your own home. Be proactive by not stocking your favorite indulgences in the kitchen.

When you have the urge to sneak a few bites of ice cream before bed, you'll be unable to do so if there isn't any ice cream to be found. Be careful not to fall into the trap of "buying it for the kids," as this is a slippery slope.

No one in the family benefits from having junk food stocked in the house. Get it out.

Step #5: Exercise Regularly

How can exercising regularly help you overcome closet eating? It's simple. When you are actively working towards a goal, and are supported, you'll be less likely to self-sabotage.

My fitness plans are designed to get you to your desired weight loss goal quickly and efficiently. There's accountability, encouragement, and measurable results to keep you on track.

Closet eating may be your way of dealing with the stress you have in your life, but you can change that. Exercise is an even more effective stress reliever.

Visit your local Fit Body Boot Camp location for a stress-busting, fat burning workout.

To Snack or Not To Snack

When you find yourself reaching for a snack—WAIT! Are you really even hungry? Or are you simply snacking out of habit?

Next time you find yourself gravitating toward a junk food fix, do a short burst of physical activity like a dozen jumping jacks and/or 15 crunches and then ask yourself if you really need those extra calories.

Ready to raid your pantry? Come, it's fun…

CHAPTER SIX

Step #5 - How to Give Yourself a Proper Pantry Raid

** Don't skip this section!!!!! **

This is one of the most important steps to ensure your fat loss success – seriously.

Completing your pantry raid is crucial to creating an environment of success.

Your Self-Guided Kitchen Raid

Your kitchen will make or break your weight loss results.

A kitchen stocked with the makings for healthy meals and snacks will keep you on track even when late-night cravings strike. On the flip side, a kitchen filled with unhealthy munchies will derail your weight loss efforts every single time.

So what should your cupboards hold and what should be off limits? I've designed this self-guided kitchen raid to help you sort out the good from the bad.

Go ahead, grab a garbage bag, print out the list below, and then head to the kitchen.

The Refrigerator: Let's start with the fridge, the heart of your kitchen. If you find something in your fridge that is on the "Dump this" list, then you know what you have to do. Get that garbage bag ready.

Dump this: **Beverages with high fructose corn syrup or sugar**. Drinking calories is one of the quickest ways to gain weight, so quickly rid your fridge of any beverage that lists HFCS or sugar on the ingredient list.

Replace with: **Water.** It is a well known fact that most people are partially dehydrated, a condition that is harmful to your health and wreaks havoc on your weight loss efforts. Keep plenty of cold water on hand for proper hydration.

Dump this: **Rich dairy products.** I know that cream cheese tastes amazing, but fat-filled dairy products are extremely high in calories and should not reside in your fridge. Eliminate high-fat cheese, milk, and yogurt from your kitchen.

Replace with: **Fresh Vegetabls.** The produce drawer in your fridge should be overflowing with colorful nutrient-rich veggies. In fact, your fridge should hold more veggies than the drawer can hold. Veggies are filled with fiber, vitamins, and nutrients and are a vital part of a healthy well-rounded diet.

Dump this: **Fatty meats.** It is important that you be selective about the meats you eat. I may tell you chicken is a great source of protein, but if you take that as a license to eat fried chicken everyday then the benefit of the protein will be lost in all the extra fat calories.

Replace with: **Lean meats.** Skinless chicken breast, lean ground turkey, white fish – there are numerous choices when it comes to lean meats.

Dump this: **Fruit-flavored yogurt.** I hate to break this to you, but that cute individually packaged yogurt is going to do more harm to your waistline than you think. More than 50% of the calories in fruit-flavored yogurt come from sugar. Check out the ingredient list and you'll likely find both high fructose corn syrup AND sugar.

Replace with: **Plain low-fat yogurt, Greek yogurt, or low-fat cottage cheese.** If you love yogurt, then get the low-fat plain version. You can even chop up some fresh fruit and stir it in. Another option is to have a scoop of low-fat cottage cheese with chopped fruit on top.

The Freezer: Next let's take a look into your freezer. Anyone who has walked the freezer aisles at the store knows how plentiful frozen temptations are. How does your freezer measure up?

Dump this: **Ice cream.** We may as well get this one over with. Hiding a gallon or two (or even a pint) of your favorite ice cream "for a rainy day" is NOT a good idea. Save yourself from that temptation and don't buy ice cream.

Replace with: **Frozen fruit.** When your sweet tooth starts acting up, throw an assortment of frozen fruit into the blender and whip up a healthy fiber-filled smoothie.

Dump this: **Frozen Pizza.** This is another one of those items that is just too tempting to keep around. Why would you bother to make a healthy dinner when a frozen pizza is calling your name? Ban frozen pizza from your home and watch as your waist starts to shrink.

Replace with: **Turkey or Veggie Patties.** For quick dinners keep your freezer filled with lean turkey patties and veggie patties. Serve on a bed of brown rice or on a whole grain bun.

Dump this: **TV Dinners.** I doubt that you need me to go into too much detail on this one. The next time you are tempted to buy a pre-packaged frozen meal, please turn the package over and read the nutritional facts. You will be shocked by the staggering number of calories and less-than-healthy ingredients.

Replace with: **Home-made Portioned Meals.** Spend some time on the weekends to cook up healthy meals, and then freeze them in portioned containers. Then throughout the week you simply need to reheat and enjoy.

Dump this: **Frozen Breakfast Food.** French toast, waffles and pancakes are popular items in the freezer aisle. Don't fall for the pretty photos and tasty-sounding names. These items are highly processed and contain loads of unnecessary sugar.

Replace with: **Sprouted Whole Grain Bread and Muffins.** It is just as easy to throw a slice of sprouted, whole grain bread into the toaster as it is a frozen waffle. Spread it with some natural peanut butter and pair it with a piece of fruit. Now that's a much healthier breakfast.

The Pantry: Last, but not least, we come to your pantry. This may be the most painful part of your kitchen raid, since most junk food ends up here. So take a moment to give yourself a pep talk before grabbing that garbage bag and opening your pantry.

Dump this: **Sugar-filled cereal.** If sugar or high fructose corn syrup are listed as ingredients on your cereal box, it's got to go. Sugar-filled cereal is basically another form of junk food, and will only add inches to your waist.

Replace with: **Whole Grain Oatmeal.** There is a huge difference between instant, sugar-filled oatmeal and whole grain oatmeal.

Dump this: **Refined/White Bread/Rice/Pasta.** These highly processed products promote weight gain and a plethora of other health problems. Do not buy "white" bread, rice or pasta – especially if you want to lose weight.

Replace with: **Whole Grain Bread/Rice/Pasta.** Whole grain is the best choice you can make. It is filled with healthy fiber and is less likely to contain harmful, waist-expanding ingredients.

Dump this: **Chips/Crackers.** While refined chips and crackers are fun to munch on, the extra calories will quickly add up. Do yourself a favor by not allowing these into your pantry.

Replace with: **Almonds.** The key to making this snack a winner is to practice portion control. Place a handful of almonds into individual bags for pre-portioned snacks.

Dump this: **Packaged Sweets.** I don't really have to explain this one, do I? Cookies, cakes, and candies shouldn't be a regular part of your diet, so keep them out of your house. It's one thing to enjoy a dessert once in a while; it is quite another to routinely eat processed sweets at home.

Replace with: **Dried Fruit.** When you want to munch on something sweet, turn to a bag of dried fruit. Make sure you purchase dried fruit that does not contained added sugars.

That completes your self-guided kitchen raid. I encourage you to raid your kitchen every couple of months as a way of keeping yourself on track. Talk with your family members about the healthy changes that you're making, and try to get everyone's support.

Shop Your Way Thin

Here's your grocery shopping cheat-sheet. Take this with you as a reminder of what to buy and what not to buy.

Don't buy food items that:

Are filled with sugar or high fructose corn syrup.

Are highly processed and contain unidentifiable ingredients.

Are full of fat.

Do buy:

Whole, fresh fruits and vegetables.

Whole grains.

Lean proteins.

Go FITNESS Shopping

Did you know that the grocery store is the source for most of your unwanted pounds?

Well, that and the fast food restaurants, but we all know that, right?

If you're like most people then your shopping trips aren't exactly organized. In fact, your grocery cart is likely to be more fat than fit.

The good news is that with a few small modifications to your routine you'll be able to turn your grocery shopping trip into an easy opportunity to slim down.

I've broken down the process of healthy grocery store navigation with an easy-to-remember acronym—FITNESS.

Come take a walk with me through your grocery store and we'll improve your shape and the shape of your family members.

F: First Veggies

Your mom always told you that you had to eat your veggies before dessert—so this will be an easy one to remember. When you start shopping, first go to the produce section. The bulk of your shopping should take place here. Fresh vegetables, lettuce for salads, and fruits are the best things to eat when you want to look and feel great.

Don't skimp on produce—aim to fill most of your cart here.

I: Is it Wheat?

When it comes to bread you only need to ask yourself one question. Is it wheat? White bread products have been processed and filled with simple carbohydrates – these will easily stick to your body as fat.

Wheat breads, on the other hand, contain more fiber and are much healthier. Make it a policy to never purchase white bread. Wheat bread is the right choice even for the little members of your family.

Always choose hearty wheat bread products—the more whole grain, the better.

T: Trim the Fat

In the meat section you are faced with a major decision. Do you go with your taste buds or do you go with your health conscious side? I urge you to stick with the latter.

These days, lean meats are more available than ever and the benefits of eating lean are numerous. When you choose lean meats you avoid extra saturated fat (your heart will thank you for this) and you also avoid the extra calories that come packed into each fat gram.

Want to be lean? Then eat lean meats.

N: Never enter the Junk Food Aisle

I have a simple policy that has saved me from thousands of unnecessary calories. I don't walk down the junk food aisle. You and I both know that it is nearly impossible to walk past rows of chips, candies, and cookies without putting something into the cart. The bright packages stamped with mouthwatering images will give your willpower a run for its money.

My two cents - Avoid that row altogether and save yourself from the whole ordeal.

Nothing good ever came from walking down the junk food aisle—just say no.

E: Edge around the store

Here's a really easy trick for healthy shopping. Edge around the store, as in shop the perimeter and avoid the inner aisles. Think about it—the healthiest products are kept around the perimeter of the store: produce, meat, dairy.

The inner aisles are where you run into trouble: processed food, baked goods, and sweets. Don't get me wrong, there are healthy products kept in the inner aisles too, but a majority of the items are waist-expanders.

Shop in a circle—stick to the perimeter of the store, do less shopping in the aisles.

S: Skinny Cow

The dairy section is filled with many healthy items; it is also filled with extremely high fat items. Your job is to pick out all those calcium-rich foods that you love in the low fat and non fat versions.

I realize that many people have a prejudice against low milk or yogurt, simply because they've always eaten the full fat version. Making the switch to low fat is such a simple way to cut unnecessary fat and calories from your diet, while still getting all the benefits of dairy.

Fat free dairy products are the way to go—you'll only lose unwanted pounds.

S: Stick with Water

Warning: mini lecture to follow. I'll make it short and sweet. Drink more water—period. Sodas, sugary juices, and calorie-laden alcoholic beverages are responsible for a large number of unnecessary calories in your diet. Don't fill your cart with these sneaky calories. Keep them out of your kitchen and out of your life.

Looking for a tasty beverage? Look no farther than crystal clear water.

There you have it—your FITNESS shopping plan that will take your cart from fat to fit. I suggest that you write down the FITNESS steps on a note card and take it to the store with you.

Are you ready to take your body from fat to fit? We've got what it takes to get you there! No guesswork, no fad diets, and no super long workouts.

Visit *Fitbodybootcamp.com* today to learn more about our fitness and fat loss programs that will quickly change your life.

Upgraded FITNESS Shopping

Want to upgrade your FITNESS shopping trips?

Here are 3 additional tips:

Don't go to the grocery store with an empty stomach. Your cart will mysteriously fill with extra unnecessary foods that will end up crashing your good intentions.

Make a list before you go to the store. You'll be able to think rationally at home before you're surrounded by tasty, FITNESS destroying foods.

Plan out your meals for the week ahead of time, then shop specifically for those items. This will cut out the junk and save you calories and money.

Now let's talk about how to order at your favorite restaurant….

CHAPTER SEVEN

Step #6 - What To Eat When Eating Out

A woman sits at a restaurant studying the menu with furrowed brow. She has begun an exercise routine and knows that her frequent meals out could slow her weight loss results if she's not careful.

When the waiter comes she is still deep in thought over what to order. "What can I get for you?" he asks with a smile. She looks up and frowns, no closer to arriving at a decision. On a whim she blurts out, "I'm trying to eat healthy but I have no idea what to order. What do you think I should eat?"

The young waiter looks startled but quickly rattles off his idea of a healthy meal. "The eggplant and roasted pepper pasta is filled with vegetables. You could get that with a salad."

The woman smiles. Yes, vegetables do sound healthy. So she orders the veggie pasta with a side salad and a diet soda, then sits back to enjoy a few slices of bread.

That's a true story. Not surprisingly the woman was unable to lose weight even though she was exercising regularly.

It is said that 80% of your weight loss results are derived from diet and the remaining 20% from exercise. So, you can see how important it is for you to stick with a healthy eating plan. This is the biggest challenge for most people especially when dining out.

When you eat at home, you know what you're getting.

Head to a restaurant and it's another story.

The ingredients, method of preparation, and portion size can easily add excess calories to your diet.

So Many Options

Restaurant menus have so many choices and are often full of unfamiliar terms. Is a food fried or baked? Does it come with a sauce or dressing? When considering what to choose from the dozens of options on the menu, you can easily become overwhelmed. It's easy to be tempted by the unhealthy choices. Just because it's on the "healthy" side of the menu, is it really healthy. Typically you won't know answers to these questions until you ask them. Don't be shy. Ask and find out what you are about to eat.

Food Preparation

Menus are often vague when it comes to the way the food is prepared. If you're not sure or the menu doesn't say how the food is prepared, be sure to ask.

Remember—restaurant foods are full of fats, as fats help keep the food moist and yummy.

To play it safe and to avoid excess fat, choose foods that are grilled, boiled, steamed, stir-fried, or poached instead of fried, baked, or battered. Also, take control of your food destiny by asking that your meal be prepared with olive oil instead of butter or other fats.

When your salad arrives, opt for oil and vinegar rather than dressing. Or have your dressing on the side so you can limit the amount you use.

Terms to watch for include "lightly breaded," "wrap," "baked," and "vinaigrette." These may all sound healthy but many are deceiving.

Foods that are lightly breaded are often deep-fried. A wrap may sound like a good option, but two slices of bread may have fewer calories than a 10-inch tortilla. Baked sounds better than fried, but it could possibly mean the food is baked deep-dish style and contains high-fat, creamy ingredients. While baked salmon is a good choice, baked lasagna is high in fat. And though vinaigrette dressing sounds healthier than a cream based dressing, it is mostly oil, so order it on the side.

Portion Control

Not only do portions keep getting bigger, so do the plates that hold them! With so much food sitting in front of you it is sometimes hard to resist the temptation to eat it all—especially when you paid so much for it.

To avoid the temptation to eat unhealthily large portions, split or share the entree, then choose a soup, salad, or extra side. If you know you'll get too much food, go ahead and ask for a to-go box when you order. That way you can divide the food as soon as you get it so you won't have to stare at the extra food as you eat.

Know What to Look For

Knowing what to look for on a menu and what to avoid will help you choose healthier, low-fat options. If you find that your diet is lacking fruits, vegetables, or whole grains when you eat out, make up for it when you eat your other meals at home.

Here are some great tips as your guide when going out to eat:

Appetizers

Appetizers are a great way to start out a leisurely meal, but can also derail your good intentions quickly.

Don't Order

Anything fried. Fried foods are a favorite but will do damage that even the most intense workout won't undo.

Creamy dips. These are filled with fat and usually come with something fried to dip in it.

Bread. It comes smothered in cheese or seeped in butter, and even when it's plain it fills you up with more carbohydrates than your body needs.

Do Order

Green salad. Ask for very light dressing (on the side) and no croutons.

Antipasto. A plate of thinly sliced meats, olives, and cheese will start you off with some protein.

Lettuce wraps. These are delicious, protein-filled and low in carbs.

Beverages

Calories in drinks are sneaky because they don't fill you up. This means that you end up taking in far more calories than you bargained for.

Don't Order

Regular or diet soda. On one hand you're drinking corn syrup through a straw, on the other you're drinking chemicals that cause you to crave sweets. It's a no win situation.

Sweet cocktails. Many restaurants are advertising sweet cocktails –resist the urge. Sugar plus alcohol equals loads of unneeded calories.

Sweetened tea. You may feel righteous for ordering iced tea, but if it's sweetened then you may as well be drinking a fully loaded soda.

Do Order

Water. Don't laugh! Water is the best beverage of all. Add a lemon for a little flavor.

Unsweetened iced tea. Don't ruin it by adding that packet of sugar. Learn to enjoy the natural sweetness to the tea.

Red wine. Stick to one glass and drink responsibly.

Entrees

This is where the real damage is done. When you order something carb-loaded you leave the restaurant feeling heavy and lethargic—you may not even realize this until you start eating better and experience the light, energetic way you'll feel after eating a healthy meal.

Don't Order

Pasta. I don't care if it comes with red sauce or white sauce, meat or veggies. If you're trying to lose weight and maintain a lean body then never, ever order a plate of pasta.

Pizza. Another dish that has far more carbohydrates than you need. If you're craving the pizza toppings then simply order those over a salad.

Burgers. If you really want a burger then ditch the bun and the fries, and have your patty wrapped in lettuce.

Do Order

Lean meat with steamed vegetables. Fish, steak, chicken, take your pick and pair it with green vegetables.

Salad with protein. Ask for dressing on the side and make sure you have a nice piece of protein on the salad.

Soup and salad. Stick with broth based soups that contain protein and pass on the breadsticks.

Adjust Your Mindset

Eating out should be a luxury, not an everyday affair. If you find yourself eating at restaurants more often than you'd like—especially if you're eating all the wrong foods, cut back on your eating out ways and watch your calorie intake drop instantly!

Your Dinner Made Healthy in 5 Steps

Do you think you're ordering healthy meals, but aren't really sure?

If your weight loss has slowed, or even stopped, then there's a good chance that you haven't been eating as healthy as you should be.

I'm going to end the guesswork for you, once and for all, with my 5 steps to a healthy meal.

By following these 5 guidelines you'll know that your meals are healthy and fitness friendly. As a result, you'll experience healthy weight loss.

Here are the 5 Steps to a Healthy Meal:

Step #1: Quality Ingredients

These are the building blocks to a healthy meal. While you certainly don't need to

dine in gourmet restaurants in order to ensure quality ingredients; you should pay attention to the quality of the foods you eat.

Choose foods that are:

Fresh and organic

Pronounceable ingredients

Whole foods

Step #2: Cooking Method

The way a meal is cooked determines how many calories, how much added fat, and the number of nutrients that survive. This simple factor will make or break your weight loss goal.

Avoid foods prepared like this:

Fried and battered

Processed and packaged

Doused with cream sauce

Sautéed

Choose foods that are prepared like this:

Grilled

Baked

Broiled

Steamed

Step #3: Mostly Protein

The bulk of your calories should be coming from a quality source of protein. With the first two guidelines in mind, these will be high quality, healthfully prepared.

Good choices of protein include:

Fish

Chicken

Turkey

Egg

Lean red meat

Beans

Step #4: Lots of Fiber

Fiber is a huge part of eating healthy and being lean. Fibrous foods will fill you up while delivering vitamins and nutrients in low-calorie packages. Fill at least two thirds of your plate with fibrous vegetables.

Try these forms of fiber:

Salad

Seasonal vegetables

Fruit

Legumes

Step #5: Lay Off the Starches

Here's where many well-meaning dieters lose it. The facts are simple, in order to maintain the low-carb, high protein diet required for healthy weight loss, there is no room for starchy foods.

Starches to Avoid:

Potatoes

Pasta

White rice and cereal

Bread and crackers

Eating Out Right

Temptations abound when you eat out. There are bread baskets, and chip baskets, and appetizers, and desserts. In order to maintain your healthy diet you'll have to have a plan in place before arriving at the restaurant.

Here's how you stay on track while eating out:

Don't eat extras: Ask for the bread basket or chip basket to be removed from your table and stick to eating only what you ordered.

Don't drink calories: Stick with water or unsweetened ice tea in order to avoid a few hundred extra calories.

Get it plain: Ask for sauces and dressings on the side to cut down calories.

Get healthier sides: Just because the grilled fish comes with a side of potatoes doesn't mean you have to get it that way. Ask for a side of steamed veggies instead.

How To Get Fat Eating at Subway

There are healthier places to eat out but done incorrectly can still cause you NOT to lose weight.

You've probably heard of Jared Fogle—he's the guy that lost over 200 pounds by only eating at Subway. His amazing story captured the attention of people all around the world. Here it is in a nutshell:

It all started March of 1998 when Jared was a college student with a problem. His weight had skyrocketed to 425 pounds. Now that's a lot of weight for anyone to handle, let alone a busy college student. So Jared made the decision to change his life.

He knew the weight would come off with the help of a healthy, low-fat diet. Luckily for him there was a Subway restaurant located near his apartment. His plan was brilliant in its simplicity. Everyday he ate the same thing:

Breakfast - coffee

Lunch - "I ate the 6-inch turkey, tons of vegetables, including hot peppers and a bit of spicy mustard." He left off the mayonnaise and cheese and had a bag of Baked Lays® potato chips and a diet soft drink

Dinner - Footlong veggie sub - again no mayonnaise or cheese.

I'm sure you know the rest of the story. The Subway diet, along with exercise, got Jared to shed the extra weight until he was a lean 190 pounds (the guy is 6'2"), and he became a spokesperson for Subway sharing his story and inspiring millions of people.

Subway then became synonymous with healthy eating.

Ever look at a Subway napkin?

It lists 7 of their sandwiches that have 6 grams of fat or less. Then at the bottom it shows you an alternative. The Big Mac and the Whopper; burgers that hold 31 and 40 grams of fat, respectively.

Wow, Subway is much healthier, right? Well, yes and no.

First read the small print. The 7 sandwiches with 6 grams of fat or less are calculated with only bread, veggies and meat. So if you take your sandwich with cheese, mayonnaise, and oil (and really, other than Jared, who doesn't?) then you need to recalculate the numbers.

Here, I'll do it for you, using a 6" Roasted Chicken Breast sandwich as an example.

Food Item	Fat	Calories
6" Sandwich (bread, veggies and meat)	6	342
Cheddar Cheese (2 slices)	5	60
1 Tbsp. Mayonnaise	12	110
1 Tbsp. Oil	15	135
Totals:	38g Fat	647 Calories

Let's not forget the tempting side items are so often picked up in the Subway line:

Food Item	Fat	Calories
Wild Rice with Chicken Soup	11	210
1oz Bag of Sun Chips	6	140
Chocolate Chip cookie	10	210
Totals:	27g Fat	560 Calories

And just like that your 'healthy' Subway sandwich grew into a meal with fat and calorie totals that rival a Big Mac meal.

Now I know you probably don't get *all* of the extras when you visit Subway but, quite frankly, that isn't the point.

The point is that there is danger in classifying any restaurant as 'healthy'.

The truth is that you could gain weight eating anywhere, just like you could lose weight eating anywhere. It all comes down to maintaining a balanced diet with a reasonable calorie and fat intake.

Jared lost weight by drastically cutting calories and fat from his diet and by starting an exercise program. You too could do this at Subway or any other restaurant. But eating at Subway does not mean that you will walk out leaner and healthier.

It all comes down to choices.

Everyday you make choices that directly affect your weight and your health. Should you get mayonnaise on your sandwich? What harm will one cookie do? Will skipping your workout today really make a difference?

You get to decide.

At some point we all reach a breaking point. For Jared, it was hitting 425 pounds. For you, it may be when you have to buy the next size up in clothing. Or when you find your body riddled with aches and pains. Or, maybe when you're shocked by the number on the scale.

Sooner or later you will decide that you *are* worth it. You will decide that your health is important. You will decide that you deserve to look great and you will do what it takes to achieve amazing results.

I want to make sure that you succeed and that's what Chapter 8 is all about…

CHAPTER EIGHT

Step #7 - How to Never Fail Again

You've come so far through this *Unstoppable Fat Loss Formula* Book, and for that you should be proud!

Right now you are pumped up and excited about turning your life around and finally achieving the body of your dreams. This is a very exhilarating place to be.

Read the following pages for tips on avoiding common mistakes that could throw you back into your old destructive habits.

5 Stupid Things Healthy People Do

You are not a stupid person. Not by any means.

In fact, it's my guess that you're healthier than most.

You probably exercise regularly. You watch what you eat. You keep up-to-date on the latest health concerns. You don't binge on sugar.

And you never – ever - eat fast food. Well, almost never.

But you do have a few unhealthy skeletons in your closet – ones that you probably aren't even aware of.

The following 5 Stupid Things are frequently committed by health conscious people. Once you break these bad habits, you'll find that achieving your weight loss goals just became a whole lot easier.

You're Dehydrated

It has been said that 75 percent of the population is chronically dehydrated. Would you disagree? When was the last time that you actually drank eight glasses of water in a day?

Dehydration occurs when more fluid leaves your body than is taken in. Symptoms include: fatigue, irritability, headaches, nausea, rapid heart rate, and, in extreme cases, even death.

Dehydration also slows your metabolism, which hinders weight loss.

You shouldn't wait until the feeling of thirst or dry mouth hits you. At that point damage has already been done. Instead, constantly rehydrate throughout your day to avoid dehydration.

The best way to do this is to incorporate water into your daily schedule. Have a water bottle at your desk and train yourself to sip on it often, and get into the habit of drinking a full glass of water with each meal and snack.

You Eat Out Too Often

Research suggests that most people eat out one out of every four meals and snacks. That's an average of once a day.

Restaurant food is designed to do one thing; to taste good. In order to increase eating pleasure, each item is loaded with fat, salt, and sugar. This causes you to eat way more calories than you actually need.

Even when you order 'healthy' items, you're still taking in more calories and fat grams than you would if you had prepared the item at home. Imagine the last salad you ordered out. Didn't it come with cream dressing, croutons, cheese sprinkles, and a piece of butter laden bread on the side?

The main reason people eat out is for convenience. So, with a little organization you'll find that preparing your own meals takes less time than you thought it would. On the weekend sit down and plan out your meals for the week. Then go to the grocery store and stock up on everything you'll need for those meals.

Pack your lunch and snacks each night before bed then grab it on your way out the door in the morning. When you prepare dinner at home, make enough for at least the next day as well. Your efforts will pay off both in terms of weight loss and in money saved.

You're Sleep Deprived

In Gallup Poll surveys, 56% of the adult population reported that drowsiness is a problem in the daytime. That's more than half of us that clearly don't get enough sleep.

Healthy adults require 7-8 hours of sleep each night. When you fail to meet this need your body goes into sleep debt, which continues to accumulate indefinitely until you catch up.

Lack of sleep negatively affects your immune system, your nervous system, and interferes with healthy hormone release and cellular repairs.

The best way to combat sleep deprivation is to set a scheduled bedtime. Your body will benefit from a consistent sleeping and waking routine and you're sure to get all the rest you need.

If you have trouble falling asleep once you're in bed, then try these two tips. First, make sure that you don't drink any caffeinated beverages after lunchtime. Second, don't eat for three hours before you go to bed. This helps eliminate sleeplessness due to indigestion and will also turbo-charge your weight loss.

You're Stressed Out

I don't have to tell you that we are living in a fast-paced world and that most of us have stress levels that are through the roof. But what you might not realize is that your stress levels are making you fat.

Stress creates an increase in the hormone cortisol and chronic stress creates a chronic increase in cortisol. This is a problem because is slows your metabolism, leads to cravings, and is linked to greater levels of abdominal fat storage.

The vicious cycle of stress and weight gain goes around and around. Stress causes you to eat emotionally and your raised cortisol levels cause that food to be stored as fat.

One of the most effective ways to instantly eliminate stress is to sit down and write out a list of all the things that are bothering you. This should include things that you need to get done, issues that weigh on your mind, and anything you believe contributes to your stress level.

Once it's all down on paper, organize it like a to-do list and start resolving each item. Doing so will get the stress off of your mind and will put your body into the motion of resolving each issue.

You're on Exercise Autopilot

You do the same thing each and every time you exercise. Same machines, same pace, same duration. While your routine sure feels comfortable, your results have long since halted.

A plateau occurs when your body adapts to your routine and weight loss stops. It is incredibly frustrating, but totally avoidable.

You don't have to increase the amount of time that you spend exercising in order to see quicker, faster results. It's all about challenging your body.

There are two simple ways to instantly increase the effectiveness of your exercise routine. First, increase your pace. Secondly, increase your intensity. Constantly vary your speed and intensity in order to keep your muscles guessing and adapting helps prevent the plateau.

Another way to break through the exercise plateau is to do something totally new. If you regularly use weight machines then start using free weights. If you normally jog on the treadmill then start using the bike.

When you join Fit Body Boot Camp your workouts are always fresh and new, always exciting, and always fun. And the best part is you don't have to figure out the routines. Just show up and do them.

5 Obstacles to Fitness Success

You want to be fit. You know how much you should weigh. You know your ideal pant size. You can even picture how great those skinny jeans will look.

So why aren't you living life in your ideal body?

There are many complex reasons that make weight loss a challenge; reasons that go deeper than simply calories-in versus calories-out.

I'm talking about the life issues that get in the way of your success.

Read the following 5 obstacles and the solutions to unlock your best body ever.

You don't want to be bothered.

It's in your DNA to avoid pain and seek out pleasure. Unfortunately, this works against you when trying to get fit. In your mind, it's painful (or at least uncomfortable) to deny yourself the tasty food that you crave and to exert yourself with exercise.

There's a simple way to work around this obstacle: Find something painful about being fat to motivate yourself towards healthy eating and exercise. Focus on the negative impact your current weight has on your health, self-esteem, and lifestyle. Convince yourself that the pain of being out of shape is much greater than the discomfort of losing weight.

You don't want to wait for the good stuff.

Just as you wish to avoid pain, you are also an expert in seeking out pleasure—namely food. This served the cavemen well, but these days it ends up as extra pounds around your waist and thighs.

There's good news - extra calories are not your only option to stimulate the pleasure center of your brain. Find an activity or two that make you smile and indulge in those regularly.

A walk outside

A good book

A night out to the movies or theater

A spa day

You can also retrain your brain to crave the pleasure of exercise-induced endorphins. Talk about weight gain kryptonite!

You are crazy busy

Let's face it, you work too much, commit yourself to too much, and don't even get enough sleep most of the time. The fast-paced way you live leaves you exhausted, stressed, and hungry for comfort food. You even begin to feel too busy to take care of your health.

It's time to reprioritize. Let go of your perfectionist standards and remove a few commitments from your schedule so that you are able to cook healthy meals, exercise, and get a good night's sleep. Remind yourself that taking care of your health is not a luxury—it's a necessity.

You don't deserve it.

I don't agree with it, but you sure act like you don't deserve to live the good life in the body of your dreams. Take a moment to think back on all the times you have self-sabotaged your weight loss efforts. If you don't believe deep down that you are worthy then you'll never give yourself a chance at a fit body.

I believe that you deserve to have a healthy body—and I urge you to dig deep down to uncover why you don't. Once you conquer your feelings of unworthiness, getting on an exercise and healthy eating plan will be easy.

Take the time to take care of yourself. You DO deserve it.

You are afraid.

You're afraid to start because you just might fail, and wouldn't that be embarrassing? You're also afraid to start because you just might succeed, and change makes you uncomfortable—even if it's change in the right direction.

When you decide to get fit you will need to go through a bushel of changes:

New diet

New exercise routine

New friends at the gym

New clothes

New self-image

Focus on all of the ways that losing weight will make your life better. Envision that better life every day so that it goes from being new and scary to familiar and comfortable.

Your friend, Regret

Have you ever felt regret the day after you passed on dessert? Of course not! You gave yourself a high-five for dodging the calorie bullet.

When temptation presents itself in the form of fattening foods or sugary desserts, decide how you want to feel the next day. Would you rather be guilt-ridden and bloated OR guilt-free and svelte?

The choice is yours.

7 Reasons Why You Can't Lose Weight

There are few things more frustrating than not being able to lose weight.

You want to be slimmer and to tone your body, but your weight won't budge.

Read the following 7 Weight Loss Blockers to discover what is standing in your way and how to quickly and easily begin your weight loss journey.

Blocker #1: Your Mind

Your mind is your number one ally when it comes to achieving your goals. However, until your mind has been programmed for success, it will do more to derail your efforts than to help you.

Take a few moments each day to visualize yourself at your ideal weight. Imagine how it feels to look the way you've always wanted.

Protect your mind from any negative self talk. If a negative thought comes to mind, immediately reject it.

You want to be thin and fit, and yet you think of yourself as out-of-shape and fat. Re-program your mind to think of yourself as fit and attractive and you will be well on your way toward achieving your goal.

Give up the belief that you can't achieve the body you've always dreamed of. See it first in your mind and then in the mirror.

Blocker #2: Your Fear

Change makes most of us nervous – even if it is a change in the right direction. You may not be consciously aware of the fear you have of getting into shape. Until you conquer this fear, your weight loss efforts will be blocked by self sabotage.

Professional speaker and author, Anthony Robbins, has outlined three specific beliefs that you must have in order to conquer your fear and instantly create a lasting change.

Believe that something MUST change. You can't be wishy-washy about it. You can't be considering it. You can't even be pretty sure about it. You've got to be rock solid about it.

Believe that YOU must change it. You can't pass the buck of responsibility and expect to lose weight. It's on your shoulders. Other people will prove to be great assets in your journey, but in the end you are the one who is going to make it happen. You have to want this weight loss enough to make it your personal mission.

Believe you CAN change it. You may have failed in the past but that doesn't matter. When you put your mind to it, you're able to do amazing things. Do you believe that you are capable of losing weight? Once you own the belief that you can, you'll be unstoppable.

Blocker #3: Your Excuses

Your excuses for being out-of-shape are getting old. An excuse takes less immediate effort than an action, but in the long run the action taker always has the advantage. Don't allow excuses to ruin your life any longer.

Don't skip out on your responsibilities with excuses; instead expect more from yourself.

Focus on the big reason why you are losing the weight. Make a list of the benefits you'll enjoy once you achieve your goal and read them first thing each morning.

Remember that you can only have two things in life: excuses or results. Which do you want?

Blocker #4: Your Commitment

How many times have you tried to lose weight only to give up a week or two later? We live in a commitment-phobic world, so it's no wonder that you routinely abandon your goals. If you truly want to lose weight then your commitment to the process is a must.

The margin between success and failure is bridged by your commitment. Don't give up until your goal has been achieved.

Treat exercise with the same importance as a work meeting and you'll never skip it at the last minute. Find three available 60-minute time slots in your schedule and mark them (in pen) on your calendar. Now stick to your schedule.

If you don't give up, then you'll never fail.

Blocker #5: Your Diet

If you consistently eat the wrong food, then you're weight loss efforts will all be in vain. To put it bluntly, you need to stop eating junk. Processed foods, refined sugar and high fructose corn syrup do not belong in your diet if you want to be in great shape. Cut these items out of your diet and replace them with real whole foods like lean meats, vegetables, whole grains, nuts and fruits.

Don't eat processed foods. Even though processed foods are accepted by our society, they contain tons of chemicals and empty calories that will make you sick and fat.

Fat contains twice the caloric density of protein and carbohydrates, so make sure to limit the amount that you consume. Eat lots of lean proteins and wholesome carbohydrates from plants and whole grains.

Vegetables, whole grains, fruits, nuts and seeds are filled with fiber and antioxidants which are vital for healthy weight loss. Snack on these instead of packaged treats.

Blocker #6: Your Patience

It takes time to transform your body from fat to fit even though you want it to happen overnight. Remind yourself that it took time to put the weight on, so it will take time to take the weight off. When you find your patience wavering or when you encounter a frustrating plateau, do the following:

Review your goal. Is it specific and measurable? Is it small and attainable, rather than monumental? Focus on your goal when the going gets tough.

Make each workout a new experience. Challenge your body with different resistance, new exercises, and a varied pace.

Remember, that anyone can have one great workout, but that won't get you the body you want. The only way to achieve your goal is by consistently exercising and eating right, plain and simple.

Blocker #7: Your Support

People who exercise alone are less challenged, less accountable, and are more likely to fail. It makes sense. Who would rush to the gym if no one is was waiting for them? Who would push themselves if no one was paying attention? Exercising alone is a recipe for disaster.

Find a workout partner who is in better shape than you, or better yet, work with me, your local fitness expert, to guarantee your results.

All of us at Fit Body Boot Camp are passionate about seeing you achieve results—don't waste your time, energy and effort on mistakes.

When you start a program with us, you suddenly have the upper hand on weight loss. I'll be in your corner, coaching you each step of the way, keeping you accountable to workouts and giving you that dose of encouragement when you need it most.

Write & Review

You could be making a valiant effort to lose weight, but if you eat too much each day then the number on your scale will not budge. Even if you think that you're limiting calories, you won't know unless you do a little research.

Get a small notebook to carry with you and jot down everything you eat for an entire week. Be sure to include the exact amount that you eat of each food item. At the end of the week do a tally of each day, and then figure out how many calories you eat on an average day. No cheating – write it ALL down.

Review your daily entries for items that are filled with empty calories – like cookies, candy, or soda pop. These should be the first things that you cut out of your diet as you transform your body.

Get to the Bottom of Your Weight Gain

Why are the numbers on your scale climbing?

That is a valid and often frustrating question. And the answer isn't always sweet and simple.

"Any change in your life circumstances can produce changes in eating and exercise, which leads to weight gain," stated Edward Abramson, Ph.D., professor emeritus of psychology at California State University and author of *Emotional Eating*.

So why has your weight increased? And, more importantly, what can you do about it?

Life's Fat Traps

A little addressed fact about weight gain is that everyone gains weight for different reasons. So often we hear about one-size-fits-all weight loss solutions that take little or no consideration of how the extra weight piled up in the first place. To experience true weight loss it is important to understand why you gained it in the first place.

Think back to the time in your life when your weight was just right. Were you in your teens? Your twenties? Or maybe your thirties? Picture yourself as you were at your ideal weight. Now, when did things change? Was it a gradual addition of pounds that accumulated over a span of multiple years? Or did you gain it all at once? Check out the following weight gain triggers and determine which one is responsible for your plight.

College: The college years are some of the easiest for gaining weight. In fact, **a recent study by Cornell University found that on average, college freshman gain about 0.5 pounds a week** - almost 11 times more than the average weight gain among 17-and 18-year olds and almost 20 times more than the average weight gain among American adults.

Marriage: There's nothing like holy matrimony to encourage a barrage of calories to overtake your diet. Late night comfort snacks are always more enjoyable when you have someone to share them with—and who better than the person who pledged to stick by your side through sickness and health?

Pregnancy: Talk about a great time to gain weight! And we're not just talking about women here. Most men admit they gained 'sympathy' pounds right along with their wife. Hormonal changes along with strong encouragement from everyone you know to indulge in anything their heart desires leave most pregnant women with a feeling of entitlement when it comes to food.

Career: Though you may not realize it, your career choice plays a major hand in your weight. Those who go from an active lifestyle to spending 8 hours a day behind a desk and another 2 hours commuting almost universally gain weight. Conversely, people who spend their 8 hours in constant motion find weight loss a natural byproduct of the job.

New Habits

Close your eyes and go back to the fat trap that triggered your weight gain. What changed your lifestyle? To help sort things out, I've broken things down into two specific behavioral categories.

Eating Habits: Did your eating pattern change at this time in your life? If your weight gain occurred in college then maybe you went from eating 3 square meals to an all-you-can-eat buffet style cafeteria. Or if marriage was your weight gain trigger, then maybe you went from eating small meals to fattening comfort food. Pregnancy brings on the perfect environment for a change in eating habits. You go from eating normally, to eating 'for two', to munching on your baby's snacks right along with him! Your job can also dictate your eating schedule. Long hours and early meetings may cause you to grab a donut or chips from the vending machine.

Activity Level: The second category that leads to weight gain is your activity level. Simply put, what kind of exercise were you doing before your life changing event and how does it compare to your current exercise regime? Chances are good that you were doing more exercise before your weight gain began—which means that you are doing less exercise today! Go ahead, think back to the exercises or physical activities that you used to do and compare them to your schedule today.

Your Transformation

You've figured out which fat trap in your life led to weight gain and then narrowed down the exact behaviors that changed as a result, so this naturally leads us to a solution.

It's time to make a change.

Don't Believe the Lies

Repetition does not transform a lie into a truth.

That bit of wisdom came from Franklin D. Roosevelt during a radio address in 1939. And though he wasn't talking about fitness, it certainly applies to the following fat loss myths.

Myth #1: Eating Late at Night Makes You Fat

The Facts: Your body doesn't have an internal timer that causes late night eats to be stored directly as fat. Weight gain happens when you eat too much and exercise too little. You could eat too much in the morning, the afternoon, or late at night and it would all result in weight gain.

Your Solution: Consider how many calories you eat and burn each day, rather than when you eat.

Myth #2: Snacking Promotes Weight Gain

The Facts: Eating snacks throughout the day is actually a great way to keep your metabolism up and to avoid overeating at meals. However, if you snack on junk food then be prepared to pack on pounds.

Your Solution: When it comes to snacking it's all about *what* you snack on. (See a list of healthy snacks on page....)

Myth #3: You Can Lose Fat Without Exercise

The Facts: Exercise and healthy eating go hand-in-hand when it comes to permanent fat loss. Your body needs exercise just as it needs to be fed a diet filled with fresh produce, whole grains, and lean protein.

Your Solution: Accept exercise as a part of your daily lifestyle. Shoot for 3 to 4 days a week of intense exercise that you can accomplish in under 60 minutes.

Myth #4: Fat Free Means 'All-You-Can-Eat'

The Facts: It's time to close your eyes and mentally erase everything that the 90's taught about fat-free dieting. Fat-free foods are not the equivalent of flavored air – they contain plenty of calories and often lots of sugar.

Your Solution: Be mindful of calories when eating fat-free foods.

Myth #5: Eat as Little as Possible for Maximum Fat Loss

The Facts: Eating too little causes your metabolism to shut down and puts your body into starvation mode and prone to store fat rather than burn it.

Your Solution: When it comes to fat loss think *burn* rather than *starve*.

Myth #6: Diet Pills Work for Fat Loss

The Facts: The only thing that diet pills are capable of burning is the extra cash in your wallet. Billions of diet pills are sold every year – all to no avail.

Your Solution: Healthy eating and exercise can never be replaced by a pill.

Myth #7: You Should Never Eat Fast Food

The Facts: It's all about what you order. Fried, processed, and salty foods will cause weight gain—don't order them. Lean meat, salad, vegetables and beans, on the other hand, are available at many fast food chains—order these instead.

Your Solution: When eating fast food skip the fried items, and stick with lean meats and salads.

Trying to lose weight is often a frustrating experience. In a world filled with quick fixes, lasting weight loss is not something that happens overnight. Remember that it took time to gain the weight, so it will also take some time to lose it.

Permanent weight loss happens as a result of a proper exercise and diet plan.

You've probably figured it out by now. *The Unstoppable Fat Loss Formula* is a **Lifestyle**, not a temporary diet and exercise plan. Move on to Chapter 9 to really understand what it means to change your lifestyle for lifelong success…

CHAPTER NINE

Step #8 - This Is Not a Diet - This Is a Lifestyle

Your lifestyle is comprised of the things that you habitually do.

What you eat regularly. How often you exercise. How intensely you exercise.

The previous chapters have given you a blueprint for a lifestyle that leads to fat loss.

Now it's up to you to make these blueprints your lifestyle…your habits.

The Habits That Make You

What are your habits?

Do you eat the same thing for lunch, go through the same exercise routine, and fall into bed at the same time each night?

Or maybe you've made a habit out of eating whatever looks good, avoiding the gym, and staying up as late as possible.

John Dryden famously said, "We first make our habits and then our habits make us."

Confucius said, "Men's natures are alike; it is their habits that separate them."

And Aristotle noticed that, "We are what we repeatedly do. Excellence then, is not an act, but a habit."

It's pretty clear that the habits you adopt will shape who you are.

When it comes to your body, the two habits that define your physique are your eating and exercise habits. In fact, everyone you know who is in great shape has dialed in these two important habits.

If you aren't happy with your body then simply adjust your eating and exercise habits. Here's how to adopt a habit:

Making a Habit

Use these seven steps to create a life-improving habit.

Decide on the ONE habit that you would like to develop. It's tempting to pick up three or four healthy habits, but choosing just one new habit is realistic and doable.

Here are some healthy habit ideas:

Do not eat after 7pm each night.

Bring your lunch to work instead of eating fast food.

Exercise 4 times a week after work for 45 minutes each time.

Only eat fruits and veggies as your afternoon snack.

Get up early and exercise for an hour each morning.

Work with a personal trainer 3 times a week.

Write your new habit down on paper. Also include your three main motivators for developing this new habit, the obstacles you'll face, and your strategies for overcoming these obstacles.

Here's an example:

My new habit is to work with a personal trainer 3 times each week.

My 3 main motivators are 1) to feel confident in my bathing suit this summer, 2) to have more energy, and 3) to fit into my skinny jeans.

The obstacles I will face are 1) not having the energy to go to my session after work, 2) not having enough money to pay for sessions, and 3) not having my spouse's support.

I will overcome these obstacles by 1) doing my workouts before work instead of after work, so I have more energy, 2) cutting down on frivolous spending to ensure that I can afford it, and 3) asking my spouse to join me so we can get in shape together.

Commit fully to your new habit, in a public way. This could mean posting it on Facebook, or simply announcing it at the dinner table. Put yourself in a position where you'll be embarrassed to give up on your new habit.

Keep track of your progress. You could keep a detailed journal or simply make a check mark on each calendar day that you successfully exercise your new habit.

Keep yourself publically accountable. This means either status updates on Facebook or verbal status updates at the dinner table. Your friends and family are in a position to offer you support, so don't shy away from those close to you.

If you fail, figure out what went wrong so that you can plan around it in the future.

Reward yourself for your success.

Once your new habit becomes second nature, usually in about 30 days, feel free to add a second habit by going through the same 7 steps.

7 Habits of Highly Fit People

These 7 habits are what separate the fit from the flabby.

Lots of people ask me how to quickly and easily get fit. While I know they are hoping for a simple answer, the reality is that getting and staying fit is a lifestyle, not a quick fix.

So what do fit people do in their "healthy lifestyle"? Take a peek with the following 7 Habits of Highly Fit People:

Habit #1: They Don't Buy Junk

Fit people know if they keep junk food in the house it will land on their waist sooner or later, so they don't buy any.

Even buying junk food for your kids or spouse is not advised since:

You'll likely eat some of it eventually

Your loved ones shouldn't be eating that junk either. It's called junk for a reason.

Rid your home of chips, cookies, candy, baked goods, pre-packaged snacks, and anything else that belongs in a vending machine.

Replace the above with fresh fruit, veggies, nuts, and other healthy whole foods snacks.

Habit #2: They Have Priorities

Fit people make exercise a priority. Along with keeping a job, paying the bills, and going to the doctor, exercise is an important part of their lives. What I've found is that fit people put exercise before leisure time. Sure, fit people enjoy leisure, but it is scheduled around their workout time.

Treat exercise time with the same importance that you would a business meeting or trip to the dentist.

Habit #3: They Stop When Full

Fit people stop eating when they feel full. Sound simple? It is, but how many times have you stuffed yourself simply to clear your plate? Or how many times have you eaten another piece of cake despite being stuffed?

The next time you feel full, take it as a sign to stop eating. Yes, even if your plate isn't empty.

Habit #4: They Push Themselves

Not only do fit people make time to go to the gym, they challenge themselves during each workout. While it is easy to simply go through the motions while exercising, you're cheating your body out of great results when you don't push yourself.

Exercise should make you sweat, make your muscles burn, and leave you with a feeling of accomplishment.

Find ways to make each workout more challenging. For competitive people, the best way to push yourself is to exercise with a friend of similar strength. Another great way to challenge yourself is to set small attainable goals. These goals could be to push heavier weight, to sprint longer, or to do cardio at a higher intensity setting.

Habit #5: They Don't Eat and Watch T.V.

Fit people know that eating in front of the T.V. is mindless eating. When your attention is on your entertainment and not on your food you'll be less tuned in to what and how much ends up in your mouth. Eating in front of the T.V. is also very habit forming. Ever notice how you crave munchies just as a reflex of sitting in front of the T.V.?

Eat before or after your entertainment and pay attention to what and how much goes into your mouth.

Habit #6: They Drink Water

Fit people drink lots of water. And not just in addition to other beverages, but instead of them. Water is their main drink, while other drinks are occasional treats.

Calorie-filled drinks are one of the quickest ways to consume excess calories which quickly turn into fat.

Consider water your beverage of choice. Drink plenty of it each day and drink other beverages only a few times each week.

Habit #7: They Are Supported

Fit people don't leave their motivation to chance. They know that if their personal trainer, boot camp instructor, or workout partner is waiting for them, they are less likely to skip a workout. It is so easy to hit snooze or talk yourself out of the gym as soon as your butt hits the couch after work. Fit people take the option of missing a workout out of the equation.

Want instant support? Simply walk into your local Fit Body Boot Camp. You will gain support from fellow members as well as the qualified instructors.

I hope that these habits have inspired you to make a change for the better in your own life.

If you already do some of these habits then congratulations – you are on your way to a better body. Make an effort to incorporate the rest of the habits to take your results to the next level.

If none, or very few of these habits describe your lifestyle, then I've got good news – you now have 7 effective new habits to start that will get you some awesome results.

Don't try to tackle all 7 at once – pick one or two to add each week and gradually work up to all 7.

Be Excellent

The most important aspect in becoming and staying fit is to be persistent.

You can exercise every day for a week, but if you follow that week with a month of no exercise then you've lost all ground.

In the words of Aristotle, "We are what we repeatedly do. Excellence, then, is not an act, but a habit."

Chapter Ten

The Meal Plans

The meal plans on the following pages have all been carefully created to give you a balanced diet that's packed with lean protein, the best source of carbohydrates, fiber, and plenty of vitamins and minerals. There are three different 21-day meal plans for you to choose from, and you'll find one that will work best for you. Now, as I've told you in this book, you want to focus on a Paleo like meal plan – that's what works best.

The cavemen had it right all along.

Before we get into a brief rundown of each of the specific meal plans, I want to give you some overall information about them that will help you to use these meal plans for the best possible results. Meal plans are a tool and like all tools they need to be used properly in order to get the job done. In this case, the "job" is to get you the body you want in the least amount of time and to do it in the healthiest way possible.

This is a Lifestyle, Not a Diet

The purpose of this book is to teach you to make healthier choices and to create a better lifestyle. This isn't a diet; although the meal plans are designed to help you lose fat and build lean muscle (which will help boost your metabolism). Diets don't work forever, but a healthy nutritional lifestyle does. So don't assume that this is a temporary "thing". Instead, look at this as your new eating style…a new lifestyle.

The problem with diets is that they're focused on fast results that are usually temporary and often impossible to stick to. Most diets are destined to fail you. However, these meal plans will get you the fast results you want, but not by depriving you, cutting out whole food groups, or making you feel like you're being punished.

You don't just want fast results; you want lasting results. That means you need a plan that you can live with forever. That being said, you may change plans or add or subtract calories as your body and your needs and goals change. That's perfectly fine; each of these plans has been carefully designed for maximum health *and* maximum results.

If you need to focus on losing fat first and foremost, then choose one of the Paleo lower calorie plans. Then as you reach a healthy body fat percentage and focus on building muscle, you may want to switch to a higher calorie plan. An upcoming competition, a little vacation weight gain, or a number of other things may mean moving from one plan to another now and then.

Why the Meal Plans are 21-day Plans

There are two very good reasons why we've provided these 21-day meal plans.

First of all, behavioral experts agree that it takes 21 days to change a habit or build a new one. That's why each of these plans is for 21 days. The exception is the meal plans that are based on calorie intake.

At the end of the 21 days, your appetite and your body will have reset themselves to want and expect a healthier daily diet. You'll also have learned how to make good choices, what sensible portions are, which foods give you the most nutrition and how to combine them for maximum effect. You'll then be ready to create your own meal plans.

On the other hand, if you like the convenience and the "no-brainer" benefits of using the meal plans, there's no reason you can't continue to use them. You can go back to the start of the 21 days and start all over again or mix and match the meals to shake things up a bit.

The second reason we've given you a plan to follow for 21 days is that making a significant lifestyle change or starting a new workout program is a big change. The last thing you need is to have to do a lot of research, calculations and lists to come up with your nutritional plan. You should be focusing on your commitment and motivation, not fat grams, calories or recipes. It takes 21 days to build a habit, and after these 21 days you'll be able to make the right food choices moving forward without having to follow a diet program or feel deprived in any way.

We've done all of that for you, so that you can direct all of your energy to working the plan, not creating it. Your attention should be on your workouts, your form and the awesome results of your hard work.

There's a Reason for Keeping It Simple

You'll notice there aren't a lot of complicated, gourmet recipes or weird, hard-to-find foods on these meal plans. Again, we want your attention to be focused in the right direction. But we also want these meals plans to be workable for anyone, whether you like to cook or can barely boil water, whether you have time to do a lot of prep or can barely manage the time to eat.

You can get fancy with the recipes later on once you've relearned how to eat and get your body to fall in love with healthier foods. For now, simple is better.

One Rule You Don't Want to Break

These meal plans have been carefully created to give you all the nutrients and calories you need. That includes snacks and treats. Do *not* be tempted to skip meals or snacks because you think it'll get you faster results; it won't. In fact, you could undermine your success by skipping meals. If you really can't stand peaches, then eat an apple, but don't skip the snack or meal altogether. It's there for a reason.

Now let's go over the individual meal plans so that you have an idea of what each one entails.

The 21-Day Calorie Plans

There are 3 different meal plans for you to choose from that come in 1200, 1500, 1700, 1900, 2100 and 2400-calorie plans. Your ideal calorie intake for fat loss is based on your age, weight, height, level of weekly physical exercise and goal weight. Your body requires a certain amount of calories to lose fat especially if you are burning between 600 to 1,000 during each of your Fit Body Boot Camp sessions. In order to get to your goal weight it's important that you fuel your body and not deprive yourself of vital nutrition by skipping meals or purposefully reducing your caloric intake.

If you workout at a Fit Body Boot Camp center then your trainer can help you choose the right meal plan for you. Otherwise, you can use the Daily Fat Loss Calorie Calculator available at **FitBodyBootCamp.com/MealPlans** to figure out which meal plan is best for your desired level of fat loss.

How To Burn Off Even MORE Fat In Less Time And Tone Your Muscle In The Process

If you don't follow an exercise program right now, or if you have a workout program and you're not satisfied with it, or maybe you just want better and faster results then I have the program for you. First off, you'll want to go to FitBodyBootCamp.com and find the Fit Body Boot Camp location near you and join the program. On average you can expect to burn 600 to 1,000 calories per boot camp session in under 60 minutes – that's way more than what most people burn in a one-hour workout at the gym.

The secret is in Fit Body Boot Camp's Unstoppable Fitness Formula training system. We design each workout program so that you burn maximum calories in minimum time, all while toning your muscles and increasing your body's natural ability to burn more fat. The FBBC workouts are crafted to incorporate high density resistant training (HDRT) along with high intensity interval training (HIIT) to give you the best possible results while putting your body into "after burn" – a state of increased and elevated metabolism that lasts as much as 28 hours after your workout ends. This helps you burn off more fat even while you're not working out. And since every Fit Body Boot Camp workout is created and led by a certified personal trainer you can bet that you'll be motivated and challenged throughout every workout – every step of the way.

Each plan, regardless of the number of calories, provides you with plenty of nutrition and plenty of food. The plans:

Have plenty of lean protein.

Provide sufficient carbs for energy, mainly from low-glycemic foods.

Have a good daily dose of fiber.

Provide a wide array of vitamins, minerals, and antioxidants.

The Paleo Living Plan

The Paleo living plan is excellent for rapid fat loss, for a beach vacation or a special event like a wedding or party. It's designed to promote faster fat loss by consuming proteins, healthy fats, high fiber vegetables and fruits without the processed sugary carbohydrates that cause blood sugar fluctuations, cravings and the desire to eat more carbs. By following the Paleo style meal plan you will always feel full and energized.

Encourages a higher consumption of high quality animal proteins.

Promotes the inclusion of all types of fats EXCEPT trans fats

Gets you eating 7-9 servings of fruits and vegetables per day

Easy to follow on vacation and in restaurants

The Healthy Living Plan

The healthy living plan is for those of you who like to have a variety of food choices but are still focused on losing fat. It's a semi-Paleo type of plan, in that there is plenty of protein from lean meats and plenty of low-glycemic plant-based foods. There are grains and legumes, which strict Paleo diets don't allow. They're there to provide added fiber and high-quality carbs as well as additional protein. This plan:

Is packed with lean, high-quality protein to help you feel full and energized.

Has just the right amount of healthy fats.

Has the carbs you need to power through your workouts and your day.

If flexible to fit your lifestyle at home or on the run.

The Low-Fat Vegetarian Plan

One of the problems many people have with a vegetarian diet, especially if they're just starting on a plant-based diet is that they're confused about how to combine foods and get enough protein, calcium, iron, and other nutrients that usually come from animal foods.

We've taken care of all that for you. So, if you're just starting a vegetarian lifestyle or are trying it out, you don't need to worry about an unbalanced diet. The vegetarian plan:

Combines plant foods in such a way that you get plenty of complete proteins every day.

Is loaded with fiber, vitamins, and minerals.

Includes a variety of fruits and vegetables to keep your meals interesting.

Includes dairy products, which you can substitute with things like vegan cheese or almond milk if you prefer.

Each plan provides you with specific foods to eat at all three of your meals and two to three snacks daily. As we've already mentioned, it's important for you to consume all of the food listed in each of the plans. If you miss your morning snack try to have it at some other point during the day. If you don't like one of the foods or recipes suggested, not a problem just swap it out for a healthy substitute you prefer instead.

You will notice that each plan describes the portion size and corresponding calorie amount for each food choice. Take note of the calorie amount when you want to swap or exchange the specific food for something else. Try to match up the calories of your alternative choice to ensure you stick to your daily caloric needs.

No matter which meal plan you choose, you're going to see great results. Not only will you look better from one week to the next, but you'll feel better as well. These plans will give you plenty of energy to get through your day and your workout program and you won't be hungry all day like you would on some quick-fix diet.

To find the meal plan type and calorie range that's best for you and your goals just go to **FitBodyBootCamp.com/CalorieFinder** and use to easy and automated calculator to figure out what your ideal calorie range should be to lose fat at your desired rate.

1500 CALORIE HEALTHY LIVING MEAL PLAN

DAY 1

Qty	Measure	Description	Protein (gm)	Carbs (gm)	Fats (gm)	Calories
Breakfast – Green Protein Shake						
1	Cup	Blueberries, raw	1.07	21.01	0.48	82.65
2	Scoops	Protein Powder	24.00	8.00	3.00	150.00
1	Ounce	Seeds, chia seeds ground	4.43	12.43	8.72	138.92
3	Cup	Spinach, raw	2.57	3.27	0.35	20.70
1	Cup	Unsweetened Almond Milk	1.00	2.00	4.00	40.00
1	Cup	Water, bottled	0.00	0.00	0.00	0.00
		Totals:	**33.08**	**46.71**	**16.55**	**432.27**
AM Snack – Hard Boiled Egg and Cucumber						
1	Cup	Cucumber, raw, slices	0.80	2.80	0.00	14.00
2	Large	Eggs, Organic hard boiled	12.00	0.00	10.00	140.00
		Totals:	**12.80**	**2.80**	**10.00**	**144.00**
Lunch – Open Face Turkey Sandwich						
1	Each	Apple - medium with peel	0.30	21.00	0.50	81.00
1/2	Cup, sliced	Avocados, raw, all varieties	1.46	6.23	10.70	116.80
1	Slice	Bread, Ezekiel Sprouted Grain	4.00	15.00	0.5.0	80.00
1/2	Tablespoon	Dijon mustard	0.00	0.00	0.00	7.50
2	Leaves,Outer					
		Lettuce, cos or romaine, raw	0.69	1.84	0.17	9.52
3	Slices	Tomato, sliced, organic	0.00	0.00	0.00	12.00
3	Ounce(s)	Turkey Breast slices, nitrate free	21.00	0.00	0.00	75.00
		Totals:	**27.45**	**44.06**	**11.87**	**381.82**
PM Snack – Hummus and Celery						
4	Each	Celery – raw stack trimmed	2.00	8.00	0.00	40.00
3	Each	Hummus, home prepared	2.19	9.05	3.87	79.65
		Totals:	**4.19**	**17.05**	**3.87**	**119.65**
Dinner – Hamburger on Portabella Mushroom with Yam						
1	Patty	Beef, ground, 95% lean meat/ 5% fat, patty, pan-broiled	22.19	0.00	5.11	141.04
1	Tablespoon	Dijon mustard	0.00	0.00	0.00	15.00
1	Piece	Mushrooms, whole, portabella, grilled	2.10	4.26	0.17	21.84
1	Medium	Salad – med. garden w/tomato, onion	1.95	14.25	0.60	74.00
1	Tablespoon	Vinegar, apple cider	0.00	0.14	0.00	3.15
1	Cup	Yam -baked	2.00	37.60	0.20	158.00
		Totals:	**28.24**	**56.25**	**6.08**	**413.03**
		Actual Total for Day 1	**105.75**	**166.87**	**48.36**	**1500.77**

DAY 2

Qty	Measure	Description	Protein (gm)	Carbs (gm)	Fats (gm)	Calories
Breakfast – Oatmeal Topped with Cinnamon, Nuts and Fruit						
1/2	Cup, cooked	Cereals, oats, slow cooking	2.71	11.22	1.06	64.35
1/2	Teaspoon	Cinnamon	0.15	2.70	0.10	9.00
1/2	Ounce	Nuts, walnuts, raw	2.13	1.92	9.13	91.56
1	Ounce	Seeds, chia seeds, ground	4.43	12.43	8.72	138.92
1	Cup, halves	Strawberries, raw	1.02	11.67	0.46	48.64
		Totals:	**10.44**	**39.94**	**19.47**	**352.47**
AM Snack – Apple with Goat Cheese						
1	Each	Apple, Medium with peel	0.30	21.00	0.50	81.00
1/2	Ounce	Cheese, goat, soft type	2.63	0.13	2.99	37.99
		Totals:	**2.93**	**21.13**	**3.49**	**118.99**
Lunch – Spinach Salad with Beans and Egg						
1/4	Cup	Chickpeas cooked	3.63	11.24	1.06	67.24
1/2	Cup	Cucumber - raw, slices	0.40	1.40	0.00	7.00
1	Large	Eggs, Organic hard boiled	6.00	0.00	5.00	70.00
1/3	Tablespoon	Lemon juice	0.03	0.43	0.00	1.33
1/4	Cup	Lentils, boiled, no salt	4.46	9.96	0.19	57.42
1/2	Cup, pieces	Mushrooms, raw	1.08	1.15	0.12	7.70
6	Large	Olives, (small-extra large)	0.22	1.65	2.82	30.36
1/2	Cup	Pepper – sweet bell, all colors, chopped	0.60	4.6	0.10	19.00
1	Tablespoon	Salad dressing, home recipe, vinegar and oil	0.00	0.4	8.02	71.84
3	Cup	Spinach, raw	2.57	3.27	0.35	20.70
		Totals:	**19.01**	**34.11**	**17.66**	**352.59**
PM Snack – Yogurt Parfait						
1	Cup	Blueberries, raw	1.07	21.01	0.48	82.65
5	Almond	Nuts, almonds, raw	1.06	0.99	2.53	28.90
1/2	Tablespoon	Seeds, flaxseed, ground	1.10	1.73	2.53	32.04
4	Ounce(s)	Yogurt, Greek, non-fat, plain	12.00	4.67	0.00	66.67
		Totals:	**15.23**	**28.40**	**5.54**	**210.26**
Dinner – Shrimp, Spelt Pasta, Mix Tomato, Zucchini and Oil						
1/3	Tablespoon	Garlic powder	0.47	2.03	0.03	9.32
1/2	Tablespoon	Olive oil – pure	0.00	0.00	7.00	65.00
4	Ounce(s)	Shrimp - boiled or steamed	23.68	0.00	1.20	112.00
1/2	Cup	tomato, diced	0.00	4.00	0.00	19.00
2	Ounce(s)	Spelt pasta	8.00	40.00	1.00	190.00
1/2	Cup	Zucchini	0.00	3.00	0.00	14.40
		Totals:	**32.15**	**49.03**	**9.23**	**409.72**
Evening Snack – Kiwi Fruit						
1	Fruit	Kiwi fruit	0.87	11.14	0.40	46.36
		Total:	**0.87**	**11.14**	**0.40**	**46.36**
		Actual Total for Day 2	**80.62**	**183.75**	**55.78**	**1490.39**

DAY 3

Qty	Measure	Description	Protein (gm)	Carbs (gm)	Fats (gm)	Calories
Breakfast - Toast with Cashew Butter and Grapefruit						
1	Slice	Bread, Ezekiel Sprouted Grain	4.00	15.00	0.50	80.00
1/2	Large (approx 4-1/2" dia)					
		Grapefruit, raw, pink	1.05	13.41	0.17	53.12
1	Tablespoon	Nuts, cashew butter, raw	2.81	4.41	7.91	93.92
		Totals:	**7.86**	**32.82**	**8.57**	**227.04**
AM Snack – Yogurt Parfait						
1/2	Tablespoon	Seeds, flaxseed, ground	1.10	1.73	2.53	32.04
1	Cup, halves	Strawberries, raw	1.02	11.67	0.46	48.64
4	Ounce(s)	Yogurt, Greek, non-fat, plain	12.00	4.67	0.00	66.67
		Totals:	**14.12**	**18.07**	**2.99**	**147.35**
Lunch – Pita Filled with Tuna, Feta, Veggies and Dressing						
1/2	Pita, large (6-1/2" dia)					
		Bread, pita, spelt	3.14	17.60	0.83	85.12
1/4	Cup, crumbled					
		Cheese, feta	5.33	1.53	7.98	99.00
6	large	Olives, ripe, (small-extra large)	0.22	1.65	2.82	30.36
2	tablespoon	Salad dressing, Italian dressing,	0.08	1.88	5.60	56.00
2	leaf	Spinach, raw	0.57	0.73	0.08	4.60
4	ounce(s)	Tuna, in water	20.00	0.00	1.33	120.00
1/4	cup	Tomato, diced	0.00	2.00	0.00	9.50
		Totals:	**29.34**	**25.39**	**18.64**	**404.58**
PM Snack – Hummus, Crackers and Celery						
4	Each	Celery - raw stalk, trimmed	2.00	8.00	0.00	40.00
4	Tablespoon	Hummus, home prepared	2.92	12.07	5.15	106.20
1	Each	Wasa Crackers, light rye	1.00	7.00	0.00	30.00
		Totals:	**5.92**	**27.07**	**5.15**	**176.20**
Dinner – Spaghetti with Salmon and Veggies						
1/2	Cup, chopped					
		Broccoli,	1.86	5.60	0.32	27.30
1	Tablespoon	Cheese, parmesan, grated	1.92	0.20	1.43	21.55
1/3	Tablespoon	Garlic powder	0.47	2.03	0.03	9.32
1	Tablespoon	Olive oil - pure	0.00	0.00	14.00	130.00
3	Ounce(s)	Salmon - broiled	18.81	0.00	10.50	174.00
1/2	Cup	Spaghetti, spelt or kamut	3.73	18.58	0.38	86.80
1/8	Cup	Tomato, diced	0.00	1.00	0.00	4.75
		Totals:	**26.79**	**27.41**	**26.66**	**453.72**
Evening Snack – Grapes and Seeds						
15	Each	Grapes - red	0.30	6.15	0.15	30.00
1/2	Ounce	Seeds, pumpkin raw	4.67	1.90	5.97	73.99
		Totals:	**4.97**	**8.05**	**6.12**	**103.99**
		Actual Totals for Day 3	**88.99**	**138.82**	**68.14**	**1512.88**

DAY 4

Qty	Measure	Description	Protein (gm)	Carbs (gm)	Fats (gm)	Calories
Breakfast - Cereal with Milk, Fruit and Nuts						
1/2	Ounce(s)	Almonds, raw	3.00	3.05	7.00	81.50
1/2	Each	Banana - med 8"	0.60	13.35	0.30	52.50
1	Cup	Kashi GoLEAN Cereal	13.00	30.00	1.00	140.00
1	Cup	Unsweetened Almond Milk	1.00	2.00	4.00	40.00
		Totals:	**17.60**	**48.40**	**12.30**	**314.00**
AM Snack – Apple Topped with Almond Butter						
1/2	Tablespoon	Almond Butter, raw	1.20	1.70	4.75	50.50
1	Each	Apple - medium with peel	0.30	21.00	0.50	81.00
		Totals:	**1.50**	**22.70**	**5.25**	**131.50**
Lunch – Veggie Burger in Pita						
1/2	Cup, sliced	Avocados, raw	1.46	6.23	10.70	116.80
1/2	Pita, large (6-1/2" dia)					
		Bread, pita, spelt	3.14	17.60	0.83	85.12
1	Tablespoon	Salad dressing, Italian dressing	0.04	0.94	2.80	28.00
2	Leaf	Spinach, raw	0.57	0.73	0.08	4.60
1	Patty	Veggie burgers	10.99	9.99	4.41	123.90
1/4	Cup	Tomato, diced	0.00	2.00	0.00	9.50
		Totals:	**16.20**	**37.48**	**18.82**	**367.92**
PM Snack – Kiwi and Walnuts						
1	Fruit	Kiwi fruit	0.87	11.14	0.40	46.36
1/2	Ounce	Nuts, walnuts, raw	2.13	1.92	9.13	91.56
		Totals:	**3.00**	**13.06**	**9.52**	**137.92**
Dinner – Grilled Salmon, Asparagus Topped with Feta and Oil						
8	Spears	Asparagus, baked	3.54	2.30	0.50	21.60
1	Ounce	Cheese, feta	4.03	1.16	6.03	74.84
3	Ounce	Fish, salmon, wild	21.62	0.00	6.91	154.70
1/3	Tablespoon	Olive oil - pure	0.00	0.00	4.66	43.29
1	Small	Sweet potato, baked in skin	1.21	12.43	0.09	54.00
		Totals:	**30.40**	**15.89**	**18.20**	**348.43**
Evening Snack – Yogurt Parfait						
1/2	Cup	Blueberries, raw	0.54	10.51	0.24	41.33
1/2	Tablespoon	Seeds, flaxseed, ground	1.10	1.73	2.53	32.04
1	Container (8 oz)					
		Yogurt, plain	13.01	17.43	0.41	127.12
		Totals:	**14.64**	**29.67**	**3.18**	**200.49**
		Actual Totals for Day 4	**83.34**	**167.20**	**67.27**	**1500.26**

DAY 5

Qty	Measure	Description	Protein (gm)	Carbs (gm)	Fats (gm)	Calories
Breakfast - Cereal Topped with Fruit and Walnuts						
1	Cup	Blueberries, raw	1.07	21.01	0.48	82.65
1/2	Cup	Cereals ready-to-eat,				
		KASHI GoLEAN by Kellogg	5.22	11.60	0.38	56.80
1/2	Ounce	Nuts, walnuts, raw	2.13	1.92	9.13	91.56
1	Cup	Unsweetened Almond Milk	1.00	2.00	4.00	40.00
		Totals:	**9.43**	**36.53**	**13.99**	**271.01**
AM Snack – Crackers with Cheese						
1	Ounce	Cheese, goat, soft type	5.25	0.25	5.98	75.98
2	Each	Wasa Crackers, light rye	2.00	14.00	0.00	60.00
		Totals:	**7.25**	**14.25**	**5.98**	**135.98**
Lunch – Turkey Meatballs and Lentils						
1	Cup	Broccoli, steamed	5.70	9.84	0.22	51.52
1/4	Cup	Lentils, boiled, no salt	4.46	9.96	0.19	57.42
1/4	Cup, pieces	Mushrooms, raw	0.54	0.57	0.06	3.85
1	Tablespoon	Olive oil - pure	0.00	0.00	14.00	130.00
4	Tablespoon	Tomato sauce, no salt added	0.78	4.45	0.12	22.20
3	Each	Turkey Meatballs	15.00	6.00	6.00	150.00
		Totals:	**26.49**	**30.83**	**20.59**	**414.99**
PM Snack – Yogurt Parfait						
1	Cup	Raspberries, raw	1.48	14.69	0.80	63.96
1/2	Ounce	Seeds, chia seeds ground	2.21	6.22	4.36	69.46
1/2	Container (4 oz)					
		Yogurt, plain, low fat	5.93	7.96	1.75	71.19
		Totals:	**9.62**	**28.86**	**6.91**	**204.61**
Dinner – Salmon, Rice, Eggplant Topped with Cheese						
1	Tablespoon	Cheese, parmesan, grated	1.92	0.20	1.43	21.55
1	Cup (1" cubes)					
		Eggplant, boiled, drained, no salt	0.82	8.64	0.23	34.65
1/2	Tablespoon	Olive oil - pure	0.00	0.00	7.00	65.00
1/2	Cup	Rice, brown, long-grain, cooked	2.52	22.39	0.88	108.22
3	Ounce(s)	Salmon - broiled	18.81	0.00	10.50	174.00
		Totals:	**24.07**	**31.23**	**20.04**	**403.43**
Evening Snack – Grapes and Nuts						
20	Each	Grapes - red	0.40	8.20	0.20	40.00
5	Almonds	Nuts, almonds, raw	1.06	0.99	2.53	28.90
		Totals:	**1.46**	**9.19**	**2.73**	**68.90**
		Actual Totals for Day 5	**78.32**	**150.89**	**70.23**	**1498.91**

DAY 6

Qty	Measure	Description	Protein (gm)	Carbs (gm)	Fats (gm)	Calories
Breakfast – Eggs on Toast and Fruit						
1	Slice	Bread, Ezekiel Sprouted Grain	4.00	15.00	0.50	80.00
1/2	Cup	Egg substitute, liquid	15.06	0.80	4.15	105.42
1	Large	Egg, whole, hard-boiled	6.29	0.56	5.30	77.50
1/2	Large (approx 4-1/2" dia)					
		Grapefruit, raw, pink	1.05	13.41	0.17	53.12
		Totals:	**26.40**	**29.78**	**10.13**	**316.04**
AM Snack – Cucumber and Pistachios						
1	Cup	Cucumber - raw, slices	0.80	2.80	0.00	14.00
1/2	Ounce	Nuts, pistachio nuts, raw	2.92	3.96	6.30	78.95
		Totals:	**3.72**	**6.76**	**6.30**	**92.95**
Lunch – Salmon Salad and Soup (Add extra veggies to salad)						
3/4	Tablespoon	Olive Oil, Extra Virgin	0.00	0.00	10.50	90.00
1	Large	Salad, large garden with tomato & onion	2.60	19.00	0.80	98.00
3	Ounces	Salmon - broiled	18.81	0.00	10.50	174.00
1	Tablespoon	Vinegar, apple cider	0.00	0.14	0.00	3.15
2	Each	Wasa Crackers, light rye	2.00	14.00	0.00	60.00
1	Cup	Soup, Amy's Organic Minestrone Soup	3.00	17.00	1.00	90.00
		Totals:	**26.41**	**50.14**	**22.80**	**515.15**
PM Snack – Apple and Cottage Cheese						
1	Each	Apple - medium with peel	0.30	21.00	0.50	81.00
1/2	Cup	Cheese, cottage, low fat, 1% milk fat	14.01	3.05	1.13	81.36
		Totals:	**14.31**	**24.05**	**1.63**	**162.36**
Dinner – Chicken, Veggies and Sweet Potato						
1	Cup, chopped					
		Broccoli, steamed	3.71	11.20	0.64	54.60
4	Ounces	Chicken breast, white meat	26.00	0.00	1.60	124.00
1	Cup	Pepper - sweet bell, all colors, chopped	1.20	9.20	0.20	38.00
1/2	Cup	Sweet potato, baked in skin, no salt	2.01	20.71	0.15	90.00
		Totals:	**32.92**	**41.11**	**2.59**	**306.60**
Evening Snack – Sunflower Seeds and Blackberries						
1/2	Cup	Blackberries, raw	1.00	6.92	0.35	30.96
1/2	Ounce	Seeds, sunflowers, raw	2.71	3.37	6.97	81.48
		Totals:	**3.71**	**10.29**	**7.32**	**112.44**
		Actual Totals for Day 6	**107.47**	**162.13**	**50.77**	**1505.54**

1500 CALORIE HEALTHY LIVING MEAL PLAN
DAY 7

Qty	Measure	Description	Protein (gm)	Carbs (gm)	Fats (gm)	Calories
Breakfast – Bacon, Eggs and Berries						
1	Cup	Blueberries, raw	1.07	21.01	0.48	82.65
2	Large	Eggs, Organic	12.00	0.00	10.00	140.00
2	Slice, cooked	Pork, cured, bacon	5.79	0.22	7.01	88.78
		Totals:	**18.86**	**21.23**	**17.49**	**311.43**
AM Snack – Apple Topped with Peanut Butter						
1	Each	Apple - medium with peel	0.30	21.00	0.50	81.00
1/2	Tablespoon	Peanut Butter, natural	2.00	1.75	4.08	47.50
		Totals:	**2.30**	**22.75**	**4.58**	**128.50**
Lunch – Veggie Burger in Pita						
1/4	Cup, sliced	Avocados, raw, all varieties	0.73	3.11	5.35	58.40
1/2	Pita, large (6-1/2" dia)					
		Bread, pita, spelt	3.14	17.60	0.83	85.12
1/3	Tablespoon	Garlic powder	0.47	2.03	0.03	9.32
1/2	Cup, pieces	Mushrooms, raw	1.08	1.15	0.12	7.70
1/2	Tablespoon	Olive oil - pure	0.00	0.00	7.00	65.00
2	Tablespoon	Onion - chopped	0.20	1.80	0.00	8.00
1	Patty	Veggie burgers	10.99	9.99	4.41	123.90
		Totals:	**16.60**	**35.68**	**17.75**	**357.44**
PM Snack – Nuts and Veggie						
8	Almond	Nuts, almonds, raw	1.70	1.58	4.05	46.24
1	Medium	Peppers, sweet, green, raw	1.02	5.52	0.20	23.80
		Totals:	**2.72**	**7.10**	**4.25**	**70.04**
Dinner – Halibut, Broccoli and Cauliflower with Rice						
1/2	Cup, chopped					
		Broccoli, steamed	1.86	5.60	0.32	27.30
1/2	Cup (1" pieces)					
		Cauliflower, steamed	1.14	2.55	0.28	14.26
4.5	Ounce	Fish, halibut, Pacific	34.03	0.00	3.75	178.50
1	Tablespoon	Olive oil - pure	0.00	0.00	14.00	130.00
1/2	Cup	Rice, brown, long-grain, cooked	2.52	22.39	0.88	108.22
		Totals:	**39.54**	**30.53**	**19.22**	**458.28**
Evening Snack – Yogurt Parfait						
1/2	Cup	Raspberries, raw	0.74	7.34	0.40	31.98
1/2	Tablespoon	Seeds, flaxseed, ground	1.10	1.73	2.53	32.04
1	Container (8 oz)					
		Yogurt, plain	13.01	17.43	0.41	127.12
		Totals:	**14.84**	**26.51**	**3.34**	**191.14**
		Actual Totals for Day 7	**94.87**	**143.81**	**66.62**	**1516.84**

DAY 8

Qty	Measure	Description	Protein (gm)	Carbs (gm)	Fats (gm)	Calories
Breakfast –Eggs, Nuts and Fruit						
2	Large	Eggs, Organic	12.00	0.00	10.00	140.00
1/2	Ounce	Nuts, walnuts, raw	2.13	1.92	9.13	91.56
1	Cup, halves	Strawberries, raw	1.02	11.67	0.46	48.64
		Totals:	**15.15**	**13.59**	**19.59**	**280.20**
AM Snack – Kiwi						
1	Fruit	Kiwi fruit	0.87	11.14	0.40	46.36
		Totals:	**0.87**	**11.14**	**0.40**	**46.36**
Lunch – Egg and Bean Salad						
1/2	Cup, sliced	Avocados, raw, all varieties	1.46	6.23	10.70	116.80
1/2	Cup	Beans, adzuki, boiled, no salt	8.65	28.49	0.12	147.20
3	Ounce(s)	Chicken Breast / White Meat	19.50	0.00	1.20	93.00
1	Cup	Green salad w/ raw vegetables	1.00	4.00	0.00	22.00
1	Tablespoon	Salad dressing, Italian dressing	0.04	0.94	2.80	28.00
		Totals:	**30.65**	**39.65**	**14.82**	**407.00**
PM Snack – Yogurt and Fruit						
1	Cup	Blueberries, raw	1.07	21.01	0.48	82.65
6	Ounces	Yogurt, Greek, non-fat, plain	18.00	7.00	0.00	100.00
		Totals:	**19.07**	**28.01**	**0.48**	**182.65**
Dinner – Shrimp and Spaghetti						
1	Tablespoon	Cheese, parmesan, grated	1.92	0.20	1.43	21.55
1	Tablespoon	Olive oil - pure	0.00	0.00	14.00	130.00
6	Ounces	Shrimp - boiled or steamed	35.52	0.00	1.80	168.00
1/2	Cup	Spaghetti, kamut	3.73	18.58	0.38	86.80
1/2	Cup	Tomato, diced	0.00	4.00	0.00	19.00
1/2	Cup	Zucchini, boiled, drained	0.00	3.00	0.00	14.40
		Totals:	**41.17**	**25.78**	**17.61**	**439.75**
Evening Snack – Cheese and Crackers						
1	Ounce	Cheese, goat, semi soft	5.25	0.25	5.98	75.98
2	Each	Wasa Crackers, light rye	2.00	14.00	0.00	60.00
		Totals:	**7.25**	**14.25**	**5.98**	**135.98**
		Actual Totals for Day 8	**114.16**	**132.43**	**58.86**	**1491.94**

DAY 9

Qty	Measure	Description	Protein (gm)	Carbs (gm)	Fats (gm)	Calories
Breakfast –Blueberry Smoothie						
1	Cup	Blueberries, raw	1.07	21.01	0.48	82.65
2	Scoop	Protein Powder	24.00	8.00	3.00	150.00
1	Ounce	Seeds, chia seeds, dried	4.43	12.43	8.72	138.92
1	Cup	Unsweetened Almond Milk	1.00	2.00	4.00	40.00
		Totals:	**30.50**	**43.44**	**16.20**	**411.57**
AM Snack – Cashews and Tomatoes						
1	Ounces	Cashews - raw	5.00	9.00	13.00	160.00
4	Slice	Tomato, sliced, organic	0.00	0.00	0.00	16.00
		Totals:	**5.00**	**9.00**	**13.00**	**176.00**
Lunch – Meatballs with Spaghetti Squash						
1	Cup, chopped					
		Broccoli, steamed	3.71	11.20	0.64	54.60
1	Cup, cubes	Squash, spaghetti, raw	0.65	6.98	0.58	31.31
1	Cup	Tomato sauce, no salt added	3.17	18.08	0.49	90.28
4	Each	Meatballs - see recipe	20.00	8.00	8.00	200.00
		Totals:	**27.53**	**44.26**	**9.70**	**376.19**
PM Snack – Almonds and Apple						
1/2	Ounces	Almonds, raw	3.00	3.05	7.00	81.50
1	Each	Apple - medium with peel	0.30	21.00	0.50	81.00
		Totals:	**3.30**	**24.05**	**7.50**	**162.50**
Dinner – Halibut and Veggies						
1	Tablespoon	Coconut oil	0.00	0.00	13.60	117.00
5	Ounces	Halibut - broiled	37.50	0.00	5.00	200.00
1	Cup, chopped					
		Kale, steamed	2.47	7.32	0.52	36.40
1	Cup, sliced	Mushrooms, white, stir-fried	3.87	4.36	0.36	28.08
		Totals:	**43.84**	**11.68**	**19.48**	**381.48**
		Actual Totals for Day 9	**110.17**	**132.43**	**65.88**	**1507.74**

DAY 10

Qty	Measure	Description	Protein (gm)	Carbs (gm)	Fats (gm)	Calories
Breakfast –Puff Pancakes and Apple (see recipe)						
1	Each	Apple – medium with Peel	0.30	21.00	0.50	81.00
3	Each	Puff pancakes	42.00	9.30	3.45	246.00
		Totals:	**42.30**	**30.30**	**3.95**	**327.00**
Lunch – Chicken and Bean Salad						
1/4	Cup	Avocado - pureed	1.15	4.25	8.80	92.50
1/2	Cup	Beans, adzuki,	8.65	28.49	0.12	147.20
4	Ounce(s)	Chicken Breast / White Meat	24.00	0.00	0.00	124.00
1	Tablespoon	Olive Oil, Extra Virgin	0.00	0.00	14.00	120.00
1	Large	Salad - large garden w/tomato & onion	2.60	19.00	0.80	98.00
		Totals:	**36.40**	**51.74**	**23.71**	**581.70**
PM Snack – Hummus and Celery						
6	Each	Celery - raw stalk trimmed	3.00	12.00	0.00	60.00
2	Tablespoon	Hummus, home prepared	1.46	6.04	2.58	53.10
		Totals:	**4.46**	**18.04**	**2.58**	**113.10**
Dinner – Japanese Dinner – Miso Soup, Salmon and Soybeans						
1	Cup	Miso Soup	1.00	4.00	1.00	32.00
4	Each	Salmon Sashimi	24.40	0.00	6.80	164.00
1/2	Cup	Soybeans, green, boiled, drained, no salt	11.12	9.95	5.76	126.90
		Totals:	**36.51**	**13.95**	**13.56**	**322.90**
		Actual Totals for Day 10	**119.67**	**114.03**	**43.80**	**1500.36**

1500 CALORIE HEALTHY LIVING MEAL PLAN

DAY 11

Qty	Measure	Description	Protein (gm)	Carbs (gm)	Fats (gm)	Calories
Breakfast – Eggs with Toast and Berries						
1	Slice	Bread, Ezekiel Sprouted Grain	4.00	15.00	0.50	80.00
2	Large	Eggs, Organic	12.00	0.00	10.00	140.00
1	Tablespoon	Nuts, cashew nuts, raw	1.32	2.81	3.99	49.36
1	Cup, halves	Strawberries, raw	1.02	11.67	0.46	48.64
		Totals:	**18.34**	**29.48**	**14.94**	**318.00**
AM Snack – Avocado and Peppers						
1/2	Cup	Avocado - pureed	2.30	8.50	17.60	185.00
1	Cup, chopped					
		Peppers, sweet, red, raw	1.48	8.98	0.45	38.74
		Totals:	**3.78**	**17.48**	**18.05**	**223.74**
Lunch – Turkey Sandwich and Soup						
1	Teaspoon or 1 packet					
		Mustard, prepared, yellow	0.20	0.39	0.16	3.30
1	Large (4" long)					
		Pickles, cucumber, dill	0.84	5.56	0.26	24.30
4	Ounce(s)	Turkey Breast slices, nitrate free	28.00	0.00	0.00	100.00
2	Each	Wasa Crackers, light rye	2.00	14.00	0.00	60.00
1	Cup	Soup, Amy's Organic Minestrone Soup	3.00	17.00	1.00	90.00
		Totals:	**34.03**	**36.95**	**1.41**	**277.60**
PM Snack – Cottage Cheese and Chia Seeds						
1	Each	Apple - medium with peel	0.30	21.00	0.50	81.00
1	Cup	Cottage Cheese - 1% fat	28.00	6.20	2.30	164.00
1/2	Ounce	Seeds, chia, ground	2.21	6.22	4.36	69.46
		Totals:	**30.51**	**33.42**	**7.16**	**314.46**
Dinner – Shrimp and Rice						
1	Cup	Broccoli, steamed	5.70	9.84	0.20	51.52
1/2	Cup	Brown Rice - cooked	2.45	24.85	0.60	116.00
4	Ounces	Salmon - broiled	25.08	0.00	14.00	232.00
		Totals:	**33.23**	**34.69**	**14.80**	**399.52**
		Actual Totals for Day 11	**119.89**	**152.03**	**56.36**	**1533.32**

DAY 12

Qty	Measure	Description	Protein (gm)	Carbs (gm)	Fats (gm)	Calories
Breakfast – Cherry Smoothie (blend ingredients)						
1/2	Cup, without pits					
		Cherries, sour, red, raw	0.78	9.44	0.23	38.75
2	Scoop	Protein Powder	24.00	8.00	3.00	150.00
1	Ounce	Seeds, chia seeds, ground	4.43	12.43	8.72	138.92
1	Cup	Unsweetened Almond Milk	1.00	2.00	4.00	40.00
		Totals:	**30.20**	**31.87**	**15.95**	**367.67**
AM Snack – Crackers, Goat Cheese and Cucumbers						
1/2	Ounce	Cheese, goat, soft type	2.59	0.12	2.95	37.52
1	Cup	Cucumber - raw, slices	0.80	2.80	0.00	14.00
2	Each	Wasa Crackers, light rye	2.00	14.00	0.00	60.00
		Totals:	**5.39**	**16.92**	**2.95**	**111.52**
Lunch – Chicken and Lentil Soup						
4	Ounces	Chicken Breast / White Meat	26.00	0.00	1.60	124.00
1/4	Cup	Lentils, boiled, no salt	4.46	9.96	0.19	57.42
1	Tablespoon	Olive Oil, Extra Virgin	0.00	0.00	14.00	120.00
1	Cup	Vegetables - mixed, raw	5.20	23.80	0.20	108.00
1	Tablespoon	Vinegar, balsamic	0.08	2.72	0.00	14.08
		Totals:	**35.74**	**36.49**	**15.99**	**423.50**
PM Snack – Apple and Almonds						
1/2	Ounces	Almonds, raw	3.00	3.05	7.00	81.50
1	Each	Apple - medium with peel	0.30	21.00	0.50	81.00
		Totals:	**3.30**	**24.05**	**7.50**	**162.50**
Dinner – Coconut Fish and Asparagus						
8	Spears	Asparagus, baked	3.54	2.30	0.50	21.60
1	Tablespoon	Coconut oil	0.00	0.00	13.60	117.00
6	Ounce(s)	Halibut - broiled	45.00	0.00	6.00	240.00
1	Small	Salad - small. garden w/tomato, onion	1.30	9.50	0.40	49.00
1	Tablespoon	Vinegar, apple cider	0.00	0.14	0.00	3.15
		Totals:	**49.84**	**11.94**	**20.50**	**430.75**
		Actual Totals for Day 12	**124.48**	**121.28**	**62.89**	**1495.94**

1500 CALORIE HEALTHY LIVING MEAL PLAN

DAY 13

Qty	Measure	Description	Protein (gm)	Carbs (gm)	Fats (gm)	Calories
Breakfast – Buckwheat, Kefir and Peaches						
1/2	Cup	Buckwheat groats, roasted, cooked	2.84	16.75	0.52	77.28
1/2	Teaspoon	Cinnamon	0.15	2.70	0.10	9.00
1/2	Cup	Kefir	5.50	6.00	1.00	55.00
1	Cup, slices	Peaches, raw	1.55	16.22	0.42	66.30
		Totals:	**10.04**	**41.67**	**2.05**	**207.58**
AM Snack – Hummus and Cauliflower						
1	cup	Cauliflower, raw	1.98	5.30	0.10	25.00
4	tablespoon	Hummus, home prepared	2.92	12.07	5.15	106.20
		Totals:	**4.90**	**17.37**	**5.25**	**131.20**
Lunch – Tuna Salad						
1	Tablespoon	Mayonnaise - low fat	0.00	4.00	1.00	25.00
1	Large	Salad - large garden with tomato and onion	2.00	19.00	0.80	98.00
1	Ounce	Seeds, pumpkin raw	9.35	3.81	11.94	147.99
1	Cup	Tuna Solid White in water	60.00	0.00	4.00	280.00
1	Tablespoon	Vinegar, apple cider	0.00	0.14	0.00	3.15
		Totals:	**71.95**	**26.95**	**17.74**	**554.14**
PM Snack – Apple and Cashew Nut Butter						
1	Each	Apple - medium with peel	0.30	21.00	0.50	81.00
1	Tablespoon	Nuts, cashew butter, raw	2.81	4.41	7.91	93.92
		Totals:	**3.11**	**25.41**	**8.41**	**174.92**
Dinner – Steak and Veggies						
4	Ounces	Beef, Organic Flank, separable lean only, trimmed, choice, cooked	30.67	0.00	9.33	219.87
1	Tablespoon	Coconut oil	0.00	0.00	13.60	117.00
1	Cup	Vegetables - steamed	5.20	23.80	0.20	108.00
		Totals:	**35.87**	**23.80**	**23.13**	**444.87**
		Actual Totals for Day 13	**125.86**	**135.20**	**56.58**	**1512.70**

1500 CALORIE HEALTHY LIVING MEAL PLAN

DAY 14

Qty	Measure	Description	Protein (gm)	Carbs (gm)	Fats (gm)	Calories
Breakfast – Mushroom Omelet with Cheese and Veggie Slices						
1	Cubic inch	Cheese, cheddar	4.23	0.22	5.63	68.51
1	Cup	Cucumber - raw, slices	0.80	2.80	0.00	14.00
2	Large	Eggs, Organic	12.00	0.00	10.00	140.00
1/2	Cup, sliced	Mushrooms, white, stir-fried	1.93	2.18	0.18	14.04
1	Tablespoon	Olive oil - pure	0.00	0.00	14.00	130.00
1	Small	Tomato - sliced	1.00	5.70	0.40	26.00
		Totals:	**19.97**	**10.90**	**30.21**	**392.55**
AM Snack – Grapefruit and Pumpkin Seeds						
1	Each	Grapefruit - pink or red 4" diam.	1.20	23.80	0.20	92.00
1	Ounce	Seeds, pumpkin raw	6.96	5.05	13.00	153.37
		Totals:	**8.16**	**28.85**	**13.20**	**245.37**
Lunch – Turkey Stew with Salad						
1	Cup	Turkey Stew, see recipe	13.00	30.00	9.00	250.00
1	Large	Salad – large garden with tomato and onion	2.60	19.00	0.80	98.00
1	Tablespoon	Vinegar, apple cider	0.00	0.14	0.00	3.15
		Totals:	**15.60**	**49.14**	**9.80**	**351.15**
PM Snack – Guacamole with Veggie						
1/2	Cup	Avocado - pureed	2.30	8.50	17.60	185.00
1	Cup, chopped					
		Peppers, sweet, red, raw	1.48	8.98	0.45	38.74
		Totals:	**3.78**	**17.48**	**18.05**	**223.74**
Dinner – Stuffed Meatballs with Spaghetti Squash (see recipe)						
4	Ounces	Beef, ground, 95% lean meat, 5% fat	23.98	0.00	5.60	153.44
1	Cup, chopped					
		Kale, steamed	2.47	7.32	0.52	36.40
1	Cup	Squash, spaghetti, baked	1.02	10.01	0.40	41.85
1	Cup	Tomato sauce, no salt added	3.17	18.08	0.49	90.28
		Totals:	**30.64**	**35.41**	**7.01**	**321.97**
		Actual Totals for Day 14	**178.14**	**141.78**	**78.27**	**1534.78**

DAY 15

Qty	Measure	Description	Protein (gm)	Carbs (gm)	Fats (gm)	Calories
Breakfast – Fruit and Cottage Cheese						
1	Cup	Cottage Cheese - 1% fat	28.00	6.20	2.30	164.00
1	Cup	Raspberries, raw	1.48	14.69	0.80	63.96
1/2	Ounce	Seeds, chia seeds ground	2.21	6.22	4.36	69.46
		Totals:	**31.69**	**27.10**	**7.46**	**297.42**
AM Snack – Eggs and Cucumber						
1	Cup	Cucumber - raw, slices	0.80	2.80	0.00	14.00
2	Large	Eggs, Organic hard boiled	12.00	0.00	10.00	140.00
		Totals:	**12.80**	**2.80**	**10.00**	**154.00**
Lunch – Meatball Leftovers						
4	Ounce	Beef, ground, 95% lean meat / 5% fat, raw	23.98	0.00	5.60	153.44
1	Cup,					
	Chopped	Kale, steamed	2.47	7.32	0.52	36.40
1/2	Tablespoon	Olive Oil, Extra Virgin	0.00	0.00	7.00	60.00
1	Cup	Squash, spaghetti, boiled, drained, or baked, no salt	1.02	10.01	0.40	41.85
1	Cup	Tomato sauce, no salt added	3.17	18.08	0.49	90.28
		Totals:	**30.64**	**35.41**	**14.01**	**381.97**
PM Snack – Pear and Walnuts						
1/2	Ounce	Nuts, walnuts, raw	2.13	1.92	9.13	91.56
1	Each	Pear - medium w/peel	0.70	25.10	0.00	98.00
		Totals:	**2.83**	**27.02**	**9.13**	**189.56**
Dinner – Pizza, Chicken and Salad						
5	Ounce(s)	Chicken breast, white meat	32.50	0.00	2.00	155.00
1	Large	Salad - large garden with tomato and onion	2.60	19.00	0.80	98.00
1	Slice, large	Veggie Pizza	9.16	27.48	10.99	237.62
1	Gablespoon	Vinegar, apple cider	0.00	0.14	0.00	3.15
		Totals:	**44.26**	**46.62**	**13.79**	**493.77**
		Actual Totals for Day 15	**122.22**	**138.95**	**54.39**	**1516.72**

DAY 16

Qty	Measure	Description	Protein (gm)	Carbs (gm)	Fats (gm)	Calories
Breakfast – Strawberries and Banana Protein Shake						
1/2	Each	Banana - med 8"	0.60	13.35	0.30	52.50
2	Scoop	Protein Powder	24.00	8.00	3.00	150.00
1	Cup, halves	Strawberries, raw	1.02	11.67	0.46	48.64
2	Cup	Unsweetened almond milk	2.00	4.00	8.00	80.00
		Totals:	**27.62**	**37.02**	**11.76**	**331.14**
AM Snack – Feta, Cucumber and Tomato with EVOO						
1	Cubic inch	Cheese, feta	2.42	0.70	3.62	44.88
1	Cup	Cucumber - raw, chopped	0.80	2.80	0.00	14.00
1	Small	Tomato - chopped	1.00	5.70	0.40	26.00
1	Teaspoon	Vinegar, balsamic	0.03	0.90	0.00	4.66
		Totals:	**4.24**	**10.10**	**4.02**	**89.54**
Lunch – Spicy Smoked Salmon with Crackers and Cream Cheese						
8	Medium	Carrots - baby, raw	0.00	0.00	0.00	32.00
1	Ounce(s)	Cream Cheese, Light,	3.00	2.00	5.00	60.00
4	Ounce	Fish, salmon, smoked, (lox), regular	20.47	0.00	4.84	131.04
2	Cup, Shredded	Lettuce, green leaf, raw	0.98	2.01	0.11	10.80
1	Tablespoon	Olive Oil, Extra Virgin	0.00	0.00	14.00	120.00
1	Tablespoon	Peppers, hot, chili, mature red, canned, chili sauce	0.14	0.58	0.09	3.15
1	Tablespoon	Vinegar, balsamic	0.08	2.72	0.00	14.08
2	Each	Wasa Crackers, light rye	2.00	14.00	0.00	60.00
		Totals:	**26.67**	**21.32**	**24.04**	**431.07**
PM Snack – Apple and Cashew Nut Butter						
1	Each	Apple - medium with peel	0.30	21.00	0.50	81.00
1	Tablespoon	Nuts, cashew butter, raw	2.81	4.41	7.91	93.92
		Totals:	**3.11**	**25.41**	**8.41**	**174.92**
Dinner – Kamut Pasta with Shrimp						
4	Fl. oz.	Alcoholic Beverage, wine, red, Cabernet Sauvignon	0.08	3.02	0.00	97.44
1/2	Cup, chopped	Broccoli, steamed	1.86	5.60	0.32	27.30
6	Ounces	Crustaceans, shrimp, moist heat	35.55	0.00	1.84	168.30
1/2	Cup	Kamut, cooked	5.55	26.20	0.78	125.56
1/	Cup	Tomato sauce, no salt added	1.59	9.04	0.24	45.14
		Totals:	**44.62**	**43.85**	**3.18**	**463.74**
		Actual Totals for Day 16	**106.25**	**137.70**	**51.40**	**1490.41**

1500 CALORIE HEALTHY LIVING MEAL PLAN

DAY 17

Qty	Measure	Description	Protein (gm)	Carbs (gm)	Fats (gm)	Calories
Breakfast – Greek Yogurt and Blackberries						
1	Cup	Blackberries, raw	2.00	13.84	0.71	61.92
1/3	Tablespoon	Honey, unpasteurized raw	0.03	5.19	0.00	19.20
1	Ounce	Seeds, chia seeds, ground	4.43	12.43	8.72	138.92
6	Ounces	Yogurt, Greek, non-fat	18.00	7.00	0.00	100.00
		Totals:	**24.46**	**38.46**	**9.42**	**320.04**
AM Snack – Hummus and Celery						
4	Each	Celery - raw stalk trimmed	2.00	8.00	0.00	40.00
4	Tablespoon	Hummus, home prepared	2.92	12.07	5.15	106.20
		Totals:	**4.92**	**20.07**	**5.15**	**146.20**
Lunch – Open Face Roast Beef Sandwich with Salad						
1	Slice	Bread, Ezekiel Sprouted Grain	4.00	15.00	0.50	80.00
1/2	Tablespoon	Dijon mustard	0.00	0.00	0.00	7.50
2	Leaves, inner					
		Lettuce, red leaf, raw	0.07	0.12	0.01	0.83
1	Tablespoon	Olive Oil, Extra Virgin	0.00	0.00	14.00	120.00
4	Ounces	Roast Beef, Organic nitrate free	28.00	0.00	6.00	180.00
1	Large	Salad - lrg. garden w/tomato & onion	2.60	19.00	0.80	98.00
1	Teaspoon	Vinegar, balsamic	0.03	0.90	0.00	4.66
		Totals:	**34.69**	**35.02**	**21.31**	**490.99**
PM Snack – Pear with Almonds						
1/2	Ounces	Almonds, raw	3.00	3.05	7.00	81.50
1	Each	Pear -medium w/peel	0.70	25.10	0.00	98.00
		Totals:	**3.70**	**28.15**	**7.00**	**179.50**
Dinner – Sushi						
1	Medium	Salad - med. garden w/tomato, onion	1.95	14.25	0.60	74.00
2	Each	Salmon Sashimi	12.20	0.00	3.40	82.00
6	Pack	Spicy Salmon Rolls 6 pieces	9.00	46.50	3.40	248.00
1	Teaspoon	Vinegar, apple cider	0.00	0.05	0.00	1.05
		Totals:	**23.15**	**60.80**	**7.40**	**405.05**
		Actual Totals for Day 17	**90.92**	**182.50**	**50.29**	**1541.78**

DAY 18

Qty	Measure	Description	Protein (gm)	Carbs (gm)	Fats (gm)	Calories
Breakfast – Coconut Flour Pancakes (see recipe)						
1	Tablespoon	Almond butter	2.40	3.40	9.50	101.00
3	Tablespoon	Coconut flour	2.93	11.85	2.93	88.50
2	Large	Eggs, organic hard boiled	12.00	0.00	10.00	140.00
		Totals:	**17.33**	**15.25**	**22.43**	**329.50**
AM Snack – Greek Yogurt with Cinnamon						
1/2	Teaspoon	Cinnamon	0.15	2.70	0.10	9.00
1/3	Tablespoon	Honey, unpasteurized raw	0.03	5.19	0.00	19.20
6	Ounce(s)	Yogurt, Greek, non-fat, plain	18.00	7.00	0.00	100.00
		Totals:	**18.18**	**14.89**	**0.10**	**128.20**
Lunch – Spinach and Goat Cheese Salad						
1	Ounce	Cheese, goat, hard type	8.65	0.62	10.09	128.14
1	Large	Eggs, organic hard boiled	6.00	0.00	5.00	70.00
1	Ounce	Nuts, pine nuts, raw	3.83	3.66	19.14	188.44
4	Cup	Spinach, raw	3.43	4.36	0.47	27.60
1	Cup, halves	Strawberries, raw	1.02	11.67	0.46	48.64
1	Tablespoon	Vinegar, balsamic	0.08	2.72	0.00	14.08
		Totals:	**23.01**	**23.03**	**35.16**	**476.90**
PM Snack – Hummus and Broccoli						
1	Cup flowerets					
		Broccoli, raw	2.12	3.72	0.25	19.88
4	Tablespoon	Hummus, home prepared	2.92	12.07	5.15	106.20
		Totals:	**5.03**	**15.79**	**5.40**	**126.08**
Dinner – Steak and Cauliflower Rice (see recipe)						
4	Ounce	Beef, bottom sirloin, tri-tip steak, lean and fat, ¼ inch trim	23.56	0.00	13.82	225.67
1	Cup (1inch pieces)					
		Cauliflower, boiled, drained, no salt	2.28	5.10	0.56	28.52
1	Cup	Coleslaw, home-prepared	1.55	14.89	3.13	82.80
1	Cup, pieces	Mushrooms, shiitake, cooked, no salt	2.26	20.87	0.32	81.20
2	Tablespoon	Onion - chopped	0.20	1.80	0.00	8.00
		Totals:	**29.86**	**42.65**	**17.83**	**426.19**
		Actual Totals for Day 18	**93.41**	**111.62**	**80.92**	**1486.87**

1500 CALORIE HEALTHY LIVING MEAL PLAN

DAY 19

Qty	Measure	Description	Protein (gm)	Carbs (gm)	Fats (gm)	Calories
Breakfast – Peanut Butter Protein Shake (blend Ingredients)						
1/2	Each	Banana – medium, 8"	0.60	13.35	0.30	52.50
1	Tablespoon	Peanut butter	4.00	3.50	8.15	95.00
2	Scoop	Protein powder	24.00	8.00	3.00	150.00
1	Cup	Unsweetened almond milk	1.00	2.00	4.00	40.00
1	cup	Water, bottled	0.00	0.00	0.00	0.00
		Totals:	**29.60**	**26.85**	**15.45**	**337.50**
AM Snack – Avocado and Peppers						
1/2	Cup	Avocado - pureed	2.30	8.50	17.60	185.00
1	Cup, chopped					
		Peppers, sweet, red, raw	1.48	8.98	0.45	38.74
		Totals:	**3.78**	**17.48**	**18.05**	**223.74**
Lunch – Low Carb Noodles with Salmon and Veggies						
4	Ounces	Salmon - broiled	25.08	0.00	14.00	232.00
2	Tablespoon	Seeds, sesame seeds, whole, raw	3.19	4.22	8.94	103.14
3	Ounces	Shirataki noodles	0.00	1.00	0.00	0.00
1	Tablespoon	Soy sauce - Kikkoman 'Lite'	0.00	1.30	0.00	11.00
1	Cup	Vegetables - mixed, steamed	5.20	23.80	0.20	108.00
		Totals:	**33.47**	**30.32**	**23.14**	**454.14**
PM Snack – Apple and Cashew Nut Butter						
1	Each	Apple - medium with peel	0.30	21.00	0.50	81.00
1	Tablespoon	Nuts, cashew butter, raw	2.81	4.41	7.91	93.92
		Totals:	**3.11**	**25.41**	**8.41**	**174.92**
Dinner – Mexican Stir Fry Chicken and Black Beans						
1/4	Cup	Beans, black, boiled, no salt	3.81	10.20	0.23	56.76
1	Cup, shredded					
		Cabbage, stir fry	1.53	6.69	0.65	33.00
4	Ounces	Chicken breast, white meat	26.00	0.00	1.60	124.00
1	Teaspoon	Oil, peanut, cooking	0.00	0.00	4.00	35.36
2	Tablespoon	Onion - chopped	0.20	1.80	0.00	8.00
1	Cup	Pepper - sweet bell, all colors, chopped,	1.20	9.20	0.20	38.00
1/8	Cup, chopped or diced					
		Peppers, hot chili, green, raw	0.38	1.77	0.04	7.50
4	Tablespoon	Salsa - medium, no sugar added	0.00	0.00	0.00	8.00
		Totals:	**33.11**	**29.66**	**6.71**	**310.62**
		Actual Totals for Day 19	**103.07**	**129.73**	**71.76**	**1500.92**

DAY 20

Qty	Measure	Description	Protein (gm)	Carbs (gm)	Fats (gm)	Calories
Breakfast – Oatmeal and Hardboiled Egg						
1/2	Teaspoon	Cinnamon	0.15	2.70	0.10	9.00
1	Large	Eggs, organic hard boiled	6.00	0.00	5.00	70.00
1	Ounce	Seeds, chia seeds, ground	4.43	12.43	8.72	138.92
1	Pack	Hot cereal, organic oatmeal	4.00	19.00	2.00	110.00
		Totals:	**14.58**	**34.13**	**15.82**	**327.92**
AM Snack – Apple with Cheese						
1	Each	Apple - medium with peel	0.30	21.00	0.50	81.00
1	Cubic inch	Cheese, low fat, cheddar or colby	4.14	0.32	1.19	29.41
		Totals:	**4.44**	**21.32**	**1.69**	**110.41**
Lunch – Turkey Veggie Stew with Added Turkey and Salad						
4	Ounces	Turkey breast, white meat	26.00	0.00	1.60	124.00
1	cup	Turkey Veggie Stew (see recipe)	13.00	30.00	9.00	250.00
1	Large	Salad - large garden with tomato and onion	2.60	19.00	0.80	98.00
1	Tablespoon	Vinegar, balsamic	0.08	2.72	0.00	14.08
		Totals:	**41.68**	**51.72**	**11.40**	**486.08**
PM Snack – Grapefruit and Walnuts						
1	Each	Grapefruit - pink or red 4" diam.	1.20	23.80	0.20	92.00
1	Ounce	Nuts, walnuts, raw	4.26	3.84	18.26	183.12
		Totals:	**5.46**	**27.64**	**18.46**	**275.12**
Dinner – Fish and Vegetables						
8	Spears	Asparagus, baked	3.54	2.30	0.50	21.60
3	Ounce	Fish, whitefish, cooked	20.80	0.00	6.38	146.20
1	Tablespoon	Olive oil, extra virgin	0.00	0.00	14.00	120.00
1	Cup, sliced	Zucchini, baked	1.15	7.07	0.09	28.80
		Totals:	**25.49**	**9.38**	**20.98**	**316.60**
		Actual Totals for Day 20	**91.65**	**144.20**	**68.34**	**1516.13**

DAY 21

Qty	Measure	Description	Protein (gm)	Carbs (gm)	Fats (gm)	Calories
Breakfast – Scrambled Eggs with Spinach, Onion and Wasa Crackers						
4	Each	Egg - boiled white only	14.00	1.20	0.00	68.00
1	Large	Eggs, Organic	6.00	0.00	5.00	70.00
1	Tablespoon	Olive oil, extra virgin	0.00	0.00	14.00	120.00
1	Tablespoon	Onion - chopped	0.10	0.90	0.00	4.00
1	Cup	Spinach - raw	5.40	6.80	0.40	42.00
2	Each	Wasa Crackers, light rye	2.00	14.00	0.00	60.00
		Totals:	**27.50**	**22.90**	**19.40**	**364.00**
AM Snack – Pear with Walnuts						
1/2	Ounce	Nuts, walnuts, raw	2.13	1.92	9.13	91.56
1	each	Pear - medium w/peel	0.70	25.10	0.00	98.00
		Totals:	**2.83**	**27.02**	**9.13**	**189.56**
Lunch – Subway						
1	Large	Salad - large garden with tomato and onion	2.60	19.00	0.80	98.00
1	Sandwich	Subway 6" Turkey Breast Sandwich	18.00	45.98	4.48	280.00
		Totals:	**20.60**	**64.98**	**5.28**	**378.00**
PM Snack – Blueberries and Pumpkin Seeds						
1	Cup	Blueberries, raw	1.07	21.01	0.48	82.65
1	Ounce	Seeds, pumpkin raw	9.35	3.81	11.94	147.99
		Totals:	**10.42**	**24.82**	**12.42**	**230.64**
Dinner – Fish and Broccoli Rabe						
1	Cup, chopped					
		Broccoli rabe (see recipe)	3.71	11.20	0.64	54.60
1/2	Tablespoon	Coconut oil	0.00	0.00	6.80	58.50
6	Ounces	Halibut - broiled	45.00	0.00	6.00	240.00
		Totals:	**48.71**	**11.20**	**13.44**	**353.10**
		Actual Totals for Day 21	**110.06**	**150.92**	**59.67**	**1515.30**

Unstoppable Fat Loss Recipes

Diana Keuilian

RealHealthyRecipes.com

Breakfast

- Breakfast Bird Nests
- Egg Muffins
- Greens, Eggs and Ham
- Turkey, Apple & Goat Cheese Omelet
- Scrambled Tofu & Spinach
- Quinoa Breakfast Bowl
- Caveman Granola
- Real Healthy Fruit Parfait

- Low Carb Green Smoothie
- Creamy Fig Smoothie
- Peaches & Cream
- Low-Carb Pumpkin Muffins
- Real Healthy Pancakes
- Coconut Flour Pancakes
- Real Healthy Puff Pancake

Appetizers and Snacks

- Real Healthy Olive-Stuffed Meatballs
- Dates Stuffed and Wrapped
- Apricot Glazed Goat Cheese Gratin
- Whole Grain Bruschetta
- Real Healthy Chips and Dip
- Baba-Anoush Dip
- Sun-dried Tomato & Basil Hummus
- Roasted Red Pepper Spread

- Dressed Avocado
- Nuts Spiced and Roasted
- Amazing Savory Cashews
- Cheesy Kale Chips
- Tasty Tuna Boats
- Veggie Hand Rolls
- Fun Fruit Skewers

Salads and Sides

- Strawberry MicroGreen Salad
- Fruity Fennel Salad
- Real Healthy Tomato Salad
- Gourmet Spring Salad
- World's Best Cobb Salad

- Roasted Veggie Salad with Couscous
- Beverly Hills Chopped Salad
- Manly Man Salad
- Real Simple Fruit Salad
- Quinoa Minty Fruit Salad

- Real Healthy Egg Salad
- Creamy Tuna Salad with Apple and Cabbage
- Chicken Salad with Mango Chutney
- Tropical Chopped Chicken Salad
- Pesto Spaghetti Squash Salad
- Amazing Cauliflower Rice
- Quinoa with Basil and Almonds

- Roasted Brussels Sprouts & Caramelized Green Apples
- Garlicky Asparagus
- Sauteed Broccoli Rabe
- Favorite Green Beans
- Tender Summer Squash
- Pickled Beets

Main Dishes

- Turkey & Veggie Comfort Stew
- Okra & Carrot Stew
- Quinoa Harvest Stew
- Amazing Kale & Pinto Bean Soup
- Saffron Moroccan Stew
- Avocado Soup with Mango Salsa
- White Bean Ratatouille
- Pumpkin & Quinoa with White Beans
- Real Healthy Stuffed Eggplant
- Real Healthy Eggplant Parmesan
- Real Healthy Zucchini Cakes
- Best Spaghetti Squash Casserole
- Real Healthy Sweet Potato Casserole

- Tempeh & Veggie Stir Fry
- Teriyaki Tofu
- Moroccan Salmon with Braised Kale
- 15 Minute Tropical Fish Tacos
- Real Healthy Fish Sticks
- Mango Chutney Smothered Mahi Mahi on Sauteed Cabbage
- Agave Teriyaki Salmon
- Real Healthy Fried Chicken
- Southwest Stuffed Chicken
- Turkey-Stuffed Bell Peppers
- Real Healthy Pizza
- Garden Medley with Apple Sausage
- Apple Pork Chops

Desserts

- Real Healthy Zucchini Brownies
- Black Bean Brownies
- Skinny Lemon Bars
- Real Healthy No Bake Cookies
- Caveman Chocolate Chunk Cookies
- Andrew's Flourless Walnut Cookies
- Raw Apple-Nut Cookies
- Real Healthy Apple Pie
- Skillet Apple Pie
- Farmer's Market No-Bake Strawberry Pie
- Berry Crisp with Carmel Cream
- Guilt-Free Peach Cobbler
- Strawberry Fudge Cake
- Chocolate Dipped Bananas
- Caveman Candy
- Dark Chocolate Almond Bark
- Chocolate Lover's Pudding
- Real Healthy Strawberry Ice Cream
- Real Healthy Popsicles
- Watermelon Candy
- Easy Fruit Dessert
- Real Healthy Poached Pears

Breakfast Bird Nests

Breakfast is my favorite meal of the day (after dessert) so I'm always looking for new ways to cook up a morning feast. This recipe is surprisingly easy to throw together, has gorgeous presentation and tastes amazing. Because of the novelty of the tomato nest, the kids end up eating veggies at breakfast without even realizing it.

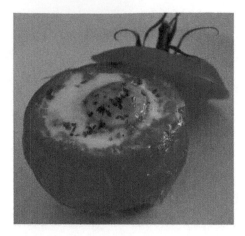

Here's what you need:

- 4 large, round tomatoes
- 1 teaspoon olive oil
- 1 clove garlic, minced (or 1 frozen minced garlic cube from Trader Joe's)
- 1 small onion, finely chopped
- 3 slices organic, nitrate-free turkey bacon, chopped
- dash of dried oregano, plus more for garnish
- dash of salt
- dash of pepper
- 4 organic, omega-3, free range eggs

1. Preheat oven to 400 degrees F.
2. Wash tomatoes, slice off the tops and scoop out the insides. Place tomatoes on a pan, and bake for 5 minutes.
3. In a skillet, heat the oil over medium heat. Add garlic. Add onion. Add chopped bacon. Saute for 5 minutes, until mostly cooked. Add the spices and mix well.
4. Turn oven to broil.
5. Fill each tomato with the bacon mixture, leaving about 1/2 inch of space at the top of each tomato. Crack an egg into each tomato then sprinkle with oregano. Place in the oven under broiler for 5 minutes. Remove from oven once the top has set, and you'll have perfectly done over easy eggs.
6. For well done eggs: change oven setting back to 400 degrees F, and continue to bake for an additional 10 minutes.

Makes 4 servings

Nutritional Analysis: One serving equals: 149.5 calories, 7.3g fat, 280mg sodium, 9.1g carbohydrate, 2.5g fiber, and 12.6g protein.

Egg Muffins

Who needs the drive-thru when you can whip up a batch of these tasty egg muffins? In the video below watch how quick and easy this recipe really is.

Get creative with the ingredients — add your favorite breakfast meat, chopped or crumbled, and add your favorite spices.

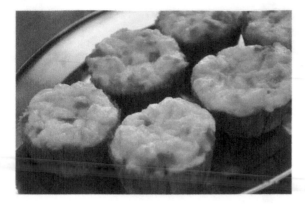

Here's what you need:

- 6 omega-3, organic, free range eggs
- 1/2 red bell pepper, finely chopped
- handful of organic shredded cheese
- sprinkle of salt and pepper

1. Preheat oven to 350 degrees F.
2. Line muffin tins with paper liners or grease with coconut oil.
3. Mix up the eggs, add bell pepper, cheese and seasonings. Fill 6 muffin tins.
4. Bake for 20-22 minutes, or until the egg is fully set.

Makes 6 Servings

Nutritional Analysis: One serving equals: 92.8 calories, 0.2g fat, 33.4mg sodium, 31g carbohydrate, 3.6g fiber, and 1.8g protein.

Greens, Eggs and Ham

Who doesn't love breakfast that comes in a cute package? I certainly do.

These Greens, Eggs and Ham cups are perfect for your healthy on-the-go breakfast!

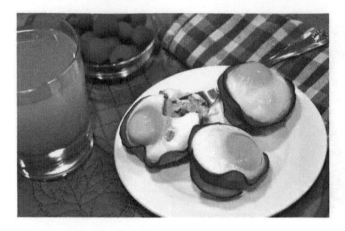

Here's what you need for 12 servings:

- 1 teaspoon olive oil
- 1 clove garlic, minced
- 1/2 yellow onion, chopped
- 12 slices of nitrate free ham
- 1 cup broccoli, steamed and chopped
- 1/4 cup shredded cheddar cheese
- dash of salt and pepper
- 12 eggs

1. Preheat oven to 350 degrees F. Lightly spray a muffin pan with nonstick cooking spray. Set aside
2. In a medium sized skillet, heat the olive oil over medium heat. Add the garlic and onions. Cook until tender.
3. Add the steamed broccoli, cheese, salt and pepper. Mix until fully combined. Remove from heat.
4. Using kitchen scissors, make a slice to the center of each piece of ham, then fold into a cone shape in each muffin cup. Fill halfway with the broccoli mixture.
5. Crack an egg into each ham cup. Bake for 16-20 minutes, or until the edges of the ham are crispy.

Makes 12 Servings

Nutritional Analysis: One serving equals: 135 calories, 8g fat, 437mg sodium, 2g carbohydrate, 1g fiber, and 12g protein.

Turkey, Apple & Goat Cheese Omelet

Omelets are one of the world's most classic breakfast foods. Don't save this recipe just for breakfast — it also makes a quick and delicious dinner. Smokey turkey bacon, cinnamon sauteed apple and creamy goat cheese create an amazing dining experience.

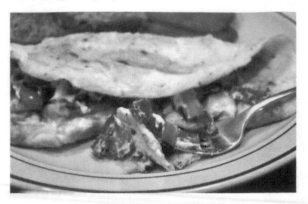

Here's what you need for 2 omelets:

- 3 slices organic nitrate-free turkey bacon
- 1 small organic apple
- dash of cinnamon
- 4 egg whites
- 2 whole free range eggs
- dash of salt
- dash of pepper
- 1 Tablespoon of unsweetened coconut milk
- 3 Tablespoons organic goat cheese

1. Place a non-stick skillet over medium heat. Cook the bacon strips for 4 minutes each side, until golden.
2. While bacon cooks, dice the apple. Remove bacon strips from skillet, place on a cutting board. Place the apple pieces in the heated skillet and saute for 5 minutes, sprinkling with a dash of cinnamon. Dice the bacon and place in a medium sized bowl.
3. In a bowl whisk the egg whites, whole eggs and coconut milk. Beat the eggs until frothy and add dash of salt and pepper.
4. Remove apples from skillet and add to the bowl of bacon. Pour half of the egg mixture in the skillet, cook until set and then flip and cook the other side. Repeat with the other half of egg mixture.
5. While eggs cook, mix the bacon, apples and goat cheese together.
6. Fill each omelet with half of the bacon, apple and goat cheese mixture.

Makes 2 servings
Nutritional Analysis: One serving equals: 249 calories, 10g fat, 485mg sodium, 10g carbohydrate, 1g fiber, and 25g protein

Scrambled Tofu and Spinach

While I don't include soy into my daily diet, once in a while a big plate of scrambled tofu really hits the spot. I especially like this version that includes spinach. Add whatever veggies you want — can't ever have too many veggies.

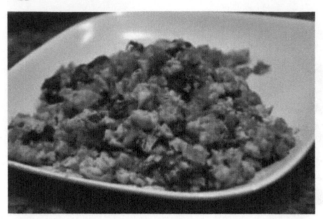

Here's what you need:

- 1 Tablespoon ground cumin
- 1 teaspoon dried thyme, crushed
- 1/2 teaspoon turmeric
- dash of freshly ground sea salt
- 3 Tablespoons water

1. Mix these ingredients together in a small bowl and set aside.

- 3 garlic cloves, minced
- 1 Tablespoon olive oil
- 1 pound extra-firm tofu, drained
- 1/2 cup nutritional yeast
- 1 cup chopped spinach
- dash of freshly ground pepper

1. In a large pan saute the garlic and olive oil over medium heat. Add the tofu, breaking it into small pieces as you drop it into the pan. Saute for 10 minutes, stirring often. Tofu should be slightly browned.
2. Add the blend of spices, mix. Add the nutritional yeast, pepper and spinach. Cook for another 5 minutes.

Makes 6 servings

Nutritional Analysis: One serving equals: 107 calories, 4.6g fat, 35.7mg sodium, 8.6g carbohydrate, 4.8g fiber, and 10.7g protein.

Quinoa Breakfast Bowl

If you haven't noticed, quinoa is the new super food. It's high in protein (12%-18%), and contains a balanced set of essential amino acids — this means it's a surprisingly complete protein. It's also high in fiber and iron. And, as if it didn't have enough going for it, NASA is thinking about growing it in space (no, I didn't make that up).

Quinoa is quite possibly the perfect thing to eat in the morning to start your day off on the right foot. And when you use leftover quinoa from the night before it is also quick to prepare.

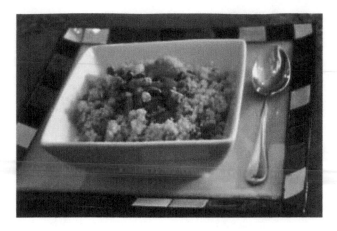

Here's what you need:

- Cooked quinoa
- Dash of cinnamon
- Dash of nutmeg
- Raisins
- Date pieces
- Pecan pieces
- Drizzle of pure maple syrup

1. Microwave your cooked quinoa for 30-60 seconds, or re-heat on the stove.
2. Mix in the spices, dried fruit, pecans and maple syrup.

Makes 2 servings

Nutritional Analysis: One serving equals: 219 calories, 6g fat, 8mg sodium, 44.7g carbohydrate, 4.2g fiber, and 7.6g protein.

Caveman Granola

Most quick breakfast foods are nothing more than grains and dairy — two things that will weigh you down rather than give you the boost of energy you need. The solution? Make enough Caveman granola to last you all week, and simply grab it out of the fridge, douse it in coconut milk and sprinkle on some fresh fruit. Now that's a quick, energy-boosting breakfast that will get your day started right.

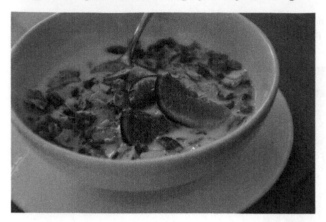

Here's what you need:

- 3 Tablespoons coconut oil, melted
- 3 Tablespoons raw honey, melted
- 1 Tablespoon vanilla extract
- 1/4 teaspoon almond extract
- 1 cup unsweetened coconut flakes
- 1 cup sliced almonds
- 1 cup pecans, chopped
- 2 Tablespoons flax seeds, ground
- 2 Tablespoons chia seeds, ground (optional)
- 2 teaspoons cinnamon, ground
- 1 teaspoon nutmeg, ground

1. Preheat oven to 300 degrees F. Lightly grease baking sheet with coconut oil.
2. Melt the coconut oil and honey together over low heat. Remove from heat. Mix in the vanilla and almond extracts.
3. In a large bowl combine all of the remaining ingredients, then mix in the coconut oil mixture until evenly coated.
4. Spread granola over prepared pan. Bake for 10 minutes, stir, and then bake for another 10 minutes or until golden brown.

Makes 12 servings

Nutritional Analysis: One serving equals: 210.5 calories, 18.5g fat, 2mg sodium, 10.5g carbohydrate, 3.9g fiber, and 3.7g protein.

Real Healthy Fruit Parfait

I'm sick and tired of fast food restaurants and coffee shops listing their fruit parfaits as the healthy option. News flash: commercial fruit parfaits are loaded with sugar and carbohydrates! McDonald's fruit parfait has 31 grams of carbohydrates — 21 grams coming from sugar– and only 4 grams of protein. That snack is going to skyrocket your blood sugar and quickly end up in added pounds. This Real Healthy Fruit Parfait recipe has 14 grams of carbohydrates and 37 grams of protein.

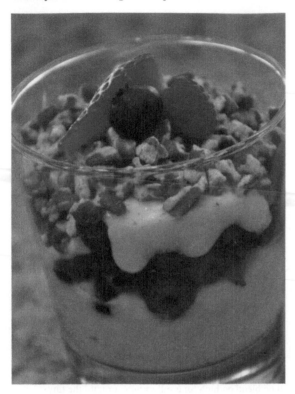

Here's what you need:

- 1/4 cup nonfat, plain Greek yogurt
- 1/4 cup lowfat cottage cheese
- 1 scoop strawberry protein powder
- 1/4 cup fresh berries
- 1 Tablespoon pecans, toasted and chopped

1. In a small bowl combine the yogurt, cottage cheese and protein powder with a whisk.
2. Place half of the yogurt mixture in a glass, top with the berries and then the remainder of the yogurt.
3. Top with chopped pecans.

Makes 1 serving

Nutritional Analysis: One serving equals: 266 calories, 7.9g fat, 303mg sodium, 15.5g carbohydrate, 2.3g fiber, and 32g protein.

Low Carb Green Smoothie

There are days that call for the cleansing power of greens –you know what I'm talking about.

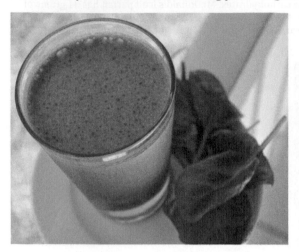

Here's what you need for 2 servings:

- 1 cup coconut water
- 1 Tablespoon almond butter
- 1/4 cup wheat grass
- 2 cups spinach
- 1 scoop high quality, low carb chocolate protein
- 1 inch slice of banana
- Optional pinch of Stevia
- 1/2 cup ice

1. Combine all the ingredients in your high speed blender then blend on high for a full minute, or until the tiny pieces of spinach have disappeared and the smoothie turns a brilliant shade of green.

Makes 2 Servings

Nutritional Analysis: One serving equals: 155 calories, 4g fat, 105mg sodium, 15g carbohydrate, 2g fiber, and 15g protein.

Creamy Fig Smoothie

I made this yummy smoothie after receiving a huge bowl of fresh, ripe figs from my mother-in-law, my favorite treat. It is packed with potassium and omega 3 fatty acids, two things we could all use more of in our diets. Also this smoothie will NOT skyrocket your blood sugar levels like most do. It's delicately sweet, creamy and very satisfying.

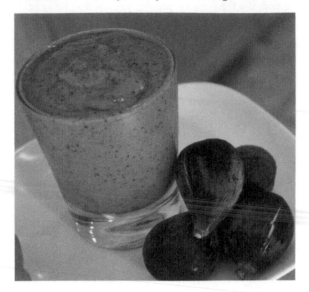

Here's what you need:

- 1 cup ice
- 1 cup unsweetened, chilled coconut milk
- 4-6 ripe figs, stems removed
- 1 date, pit removed
- 1 Tablespoon chia seed powder
- 1 Tablespoon flax meal
- 2 Tablespoons almond butter

1. Throw everything into your high speed blender and blend until smooth!

Note: It will thicken after a few minutes due to the chia and flax.

Makes 2 servings

Nutritional Analysis: One serving equals: 305 calories, 14.4g fat, 45mg sodium, 43.1g carbohydrate, 10.9g fiber, and 7.5g protein.

Peaches and Cream

This dessert requires very little preparation and tastes almost too good for words. It's a great recipe to use while entertaining, since the peaches need to sit in the dehydrator for 4 hours–put them in before your dinner guests arrive and prepare the sauce and keep in the fridge until chow time. To serve simply plate the peach halves and top with a spoonful of sauce and a sprinkle of fresh ground cinnamon. Use the sweetest peaches you can find, ripe and in season for the best possible flavor.

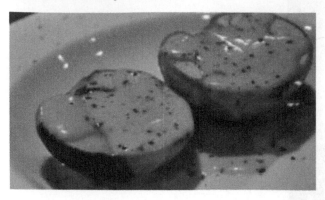

Here's what you need:

For the Cream Sauce:

- 1 Tablespoon vanilla extract (or use ground vanilla beans)
- 1/2 cup coconut water
- 1 cup pine nuts
- dash of fresh ground sea salt
- 1/3 cup agave nectar

For the Peaches:

- 6 peaches, halved
- 1/2 cup agave nectar
- 1 teaspoon ground cinnamon
- 1/4 teaspoon ground nutmeg

1. For the cream sauce: Blend all the ingredients in a high speed blender and store in an airtight container in the fridge.
2. For the peaches: Place the halved peaches on lined dehydrator trays. Combine the agave nectar and spices in a high speed blender until creamy. Spoon over the peaches. Dehydrate at 110 degrees for 4 hours.
3. Assembly: Place 2 peach halves on each plate, spoon on the cream sauce and sprinkle with freshly ground cinnamon.

Makes 6 servings

Nutritional Analysis: One serving equals: 320.5 calories, 14.2g fat, 45.5mg sodium, 40.8g carbohydrate, 3.7g fiber, and 4.5g protein.

Low Carb Pumpkin Muffins

Pumpkin has a wonderful flavor and consistency for baking, so don't limit yourself to pumpkin pie twice a year. These muffins are packed with protein, vitamins and minerals, while being low on waist-expanding carbohydrates. Enjoy with a piping hot cup of coffee for breakfast or an afternoon snack.

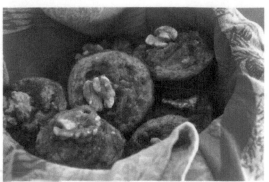

Here's what you need

- ½ cup coconut flour
- 1 Tablespoon ground cinnamon
- ½ teaspoon ground nutmeg
- ¼ teaspoon ground cloves
- ½ teaspoon baking soda
- ½ teaspoon salt
- ½ cup canned pureed pumpkin
- 6 eggs, beaten
- 3 Tablespoon coconut oil, melted
- 1/3 cup raw honey, melted
- 1 teaspoon vanilla extract
- 1/2 cup walnuts, chopped
- 12 walnuts for topping
- 1/4 cup Coconut crystals *optional*

1. Preheat oven to 400 degrees F. Oil muffin pans.

2. In a medium bowl, combine the coconut flour, spices, baking soda and salt.

3. In another bowl, place the pumpkin puree then add the eggs one at a time, mixing well after each addition. Add melted coconut, honey, vanilla, and nuts. Mix until well combined.

4. Add the flour mixture to the pumpkin mixture, blend with a whisk until most lumps have disappeared.

5. Spoon into prepared muffin pan, filling each muffin 2/3 full. Sprinkle the tops with coconut crystals and one walnut.

6. Bake for 18-20 minutes or until golden. Place on wire rack to cool.

Makes 12 servings

Nutritional Analysis: One serving equals: 176.3 calories, 10.8 fat, 136mg sodium, 15.1g carbohydrate, 3g fiber, and 5g protein.

Real Healthy Pancakes

The only way to make a lazy Saturday even more perfect is to start it with pancakes. This recipe for Real Healthy Pancakes is filled with protein and is low in carbs and sugar. Enjoy these guilt free.

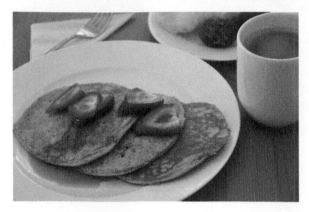

Here's what you need for 10 servings:

- 3 large omega-3, free range eggs
- 1 Tablespoon agave nectar
- 1 Tablespoon vanilla extract
- 1/2 cup filtered water
- 2 Tablespoons flax meal
- 1 1/2 cups blanched almond flour
- 1/2 teaspoon salt
- 1/2 teaspoon baking soda
- coconut oil

1. In a blender combine the eggs, agave nectar, vanilla and water. Mix until smooth. Add the flax, almond flour, salt and baking soda. Mix until well combined.
2. Grease a large skillet or pancaked griddle with coconut oil and place over medium heat. Place heaping tablespoons of batter onto the skillet and cook until bubbles form. Flip each pancake and cook for another minute, until golden on both sides.

Makes 10 Servings

Nutritional Analysis: One serving equals: 137 calories, 10g fat, 153mg sodium, 6g carbohydrate, 2g fiber, and 6g protein.

Coconut Flour Pancakes

Here's a great low carb pancake recipe. Eat these without guilt — just don't smother them in syrup.

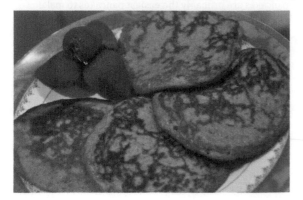

Here's what you need:

- 6 omega-3, free range eggs
- 6 Tablespoons coconut oil, melted
- 3/4 cup unsweetened coconut milk
- 1 Tablespoon raw honey
- 2 teaspoons vanilla extract
- 1 cup coconut flour
- 1 teaspoon salt
- 2 teaspoons baking powder
- 2 teaspoons ground cinnamon
- 1 cup filtered water

1. Pre-heat your pancake griddle and grease with a touch of coconut oil.
2. In medium bowl whisk the eggs, oil, milk, honey and vanilla.
3. In another bowl, combine the coconut flour, salt and baking powder. Whisk to combine.
4. Add the wet ingredients to the dry ones and mix well. Add the water and mix.
5. Cook on the pancake griddle until golden.

Makes 10 Servings

Nutritional Analysis: One serving equals: 194 calories, 13.4g fat, 267mg sodium, 9.7g carbohydrate, 4.2g fiber, and 6.3g protein.

Real Healthy Puff Pancake

Pancakes are a great breakfast no matter the weather. Puff pancakes are probably the easiest pancakes to make since you just pour all the batter into a pie pan and bake it for 20 minutes — no flipping necessary.

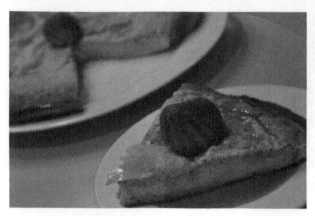

Here's what you need:

- 2 Tablespoons organic butter
- 1/2 cup non-fat Greek yogurt
- 1/2 cup water
- 6 organic, omega 3, free range eggs
- 2 Tablespoons raw honey
- 1/2 cup low fat cottage cheese
- 1 cup almond meal
- 1 teaspoon baking powder
- 1/2 teaspoon salt

1. Preheat oven to 425 degrees F. Place butter in a pie plate and melt in the oven.
2. Place all the remaining ingredients in blender and blend for 1 minute. Pour batter into pie plate.
3. Bake until puffy and golden, about 20 minutes. Cut into wedges and serve with fresh strawberries and pure maple syrup.

Makes 10 Servings

Nutritional Analysis: One serving equals: 156.2 calories, 11g fat, 203mg sodium, 7.2g carbohydrate, 1.2g fiber, and 8.7g protein.

Real Healthy Olive-Stuffed Meatballs

Lean, ground turkey, Italian seasoning and tangy olives make a winning combination.

Serve these as an appetizer, with little toothpicks, or as a main dish on a bed of spaghetti squash or sauteed vegetables. It only takes 20 minutes from start to finish.

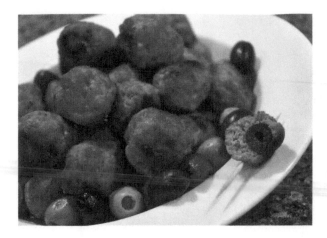

Here's what you need for 20 meatballs:

- 20 oz Italian Seasoned Lean Ground Turkey
- 30-40 pitted olives
- 1 Tablespoon olive oil
- 2 cloves garlic, finely minced

1. Take one tablespoon of ground turkey at a time, flatten it in your hand and form around an olive to create a ball. Repeat with all of the turkey and olives.
2. Heat the olive oil in a large skillet. Add the garlic and spread around the pan. Add the meatballs.
3. Turn the meatballs every 3 minutes for 20 minutes of cooking. Remove once all sides are browned and the meatballs are cooked through.
4. Serve on a platter with any remaining olives.

20 Servings

Nutritional Analysis: One serving equals: 46 calories, 3g fat, 102mg sodium, 0g carbohydrate, 0g fiber, and 6g protein

Dates Stuffed and Wrapped

With only three ingredients these dates are a quick and delicious way to impress your guests–or to treat yourself. Plump dates are stuffed with creamy goat cheese then wrapped in smokey turkey bacon. It's the perfect combination of sweet and salty. If you're not into bacon then try the variation below with dates, goat cheese and ground walnuts.

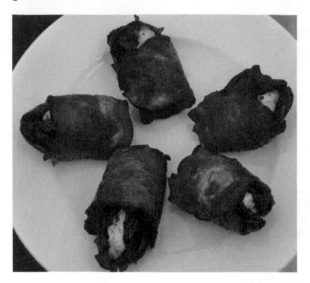

Here's what you need:

- 20 dates, pits removed
- 1/2 cup organic goat cheese, any flavor
- 10 slices uncooked organic, nitrate-free turkey bacon
- *optional* ground walnuts

1. Preheat oven to 375 degrees F.
2. Remove the pits from each date. Fill each date with a spoonful of goat cheese.
3. Cut each turkey bacon in half. Wrap on piece around each stuffed date, and secure with a toothpick through its center. Line the stuffed and wrapped dates on a baking sheet.
4. Bake for 20 minutes. Once cooked, remove the tooth picks. The bacon will maintain its shape and will hold the date together.

Makes 10 servings

Nutritional Analysis: One serving equals: 171.4 calories, 4.4g fat, 241.6mg sodium, 33.1g carbohydrate, 2.5g fiber, and 9.1g protein

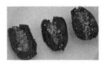 Meat free option: Stuff your dates with goat cheese and then sprinkle with ground walnuts. Bake for 10-15 minutes.

Apricot Glazed Goat Cheese Gratin

This recipe takes quality goat cheese to a whole new level by topping it with a sweet apricot crust. It's the perfect no-fuss appetizer to serve at your next party.

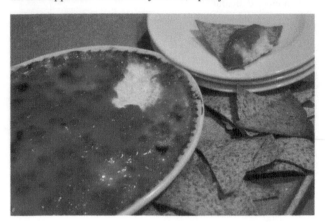

Here's what you need:

- 1 pound organic goat cheese
- 6 Tablespoons apricot preserves
- 1/4 cup pimento peppers, peeled and finely minced
- 2 teaspoons Dijon mustard
- 2 teaspoons dry sherry
- 6 sprouted grain tortillas, cut into wedges

1. Preheat oven to 400 degrees F.
2. Spread the goat cheese evenly into a gratin dish. In a small bowl combine the preserves, minced peppers, Dijon and sherry. Spread over the goat cheese.
3. Lightly grease a cookie sheet with olive oil. Scatter the tortilla wedges in an even layer over the sheet.
4. Place the gratin on the top rack of the oven and the tortilla wedges on the middle rack. Bake for 5 minutes.
5. Turn the broiler on for about 2 minutes, watching your gratin closely. The topping should be bubbly and lightly browned and tortilla wedges should be crispy.
6. Remove gratin and tortilla wedges from oven. Serve warm.

Makes 30 servings

Nutritional Analysis: One serving equals: 77.4 calories, 3.3g fat, 147mg sodium, 6.8g carbohydrate, .6g fiber, and 4.5g protein

Whole Grain Bruschetta

Who doesn't love freshly prepared tomato and basil bruschetta? While traditional recipes call for white bread, this recipe uses whole grain bread, making it healthier and even more delicious.

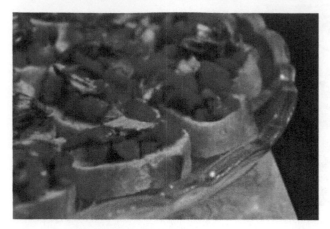

Here's what you need:

- 5 medium organic tomatoes
- dash of freshly ground sea salt
- dash of freshly ground pepper
- 1 teaspoon dried oregano
- 1 1/2 teaspoons dried basil
- 2 Tablespoons balsamic vinegar
- 12-inch whole grain baguette
- Olive oil
- 1/3 cup fresh basil leaves, chopped

1. Preheat the oven to 400 degrees. Chop the tomatoes and place in a medium sized bowl.
2. Add the salt, pepper, oregano, dried basil and vinegar to the bowl and mix well. Transfer to a mesh strainer and set it over a bowl for 12-15 minutes to drain off excess water.
3. Slice the baguette into 1/2 inch thick rounds. Lightly grease a baking sheet with olive oil.
4. Arrange the bread on the baking sheet. Brush a touch of olive oil over each slice. Bake until lightly golden, about 5 minutes.
5. Remove the bread from the oven and allow it to cool for 5 minutes, then arrange on your serving platter. Top each slice with a spoonful of the tomato mixture and sprinkle with the fresh basil leaves.

Makes 12 servings

Nutritional Analysis: One serving equals: 73.6 calories, 1.6g fat, 151mg sodium, 14.4g carbohydrate, 2.9g fiber, and 2.7g protein

Real Healthy Chips and Dip

Let's get real, as someone who takes their health and fitness seriously, fried chips are simply out of the question. So what is left to munch on at a party or while watching a movie? I'm gonna let you in on a little snacking secret of mine....jicama chips and fresh guacamole! If you've never paired these two wholesome foods then you are in for a treat. Snack away to your heart's content:)

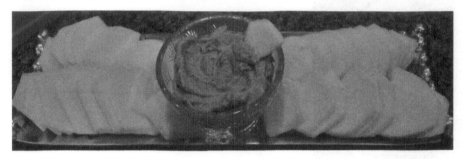

Here's what you need:

- 1 jicama for every serving
- fresh guacamole

1. Wash and peel the jicama. Cut in half and then slice into chips.
2. Serve with a bowl of fresh guacamole.

Makes 12 servings

Nutritional Analysis (with 6 oz. guacamole): One serving equals: 105.8 calories, 7.5g fat, 187.2mg sodium, 8.8g carbohydrate, 5.2g fiber, and 1.4g protein

Baba-Anoush Dip

Here is my take on Baba-Ghanoush with an Armenian flair. By the book Anoush means 'sweet', but it is also used to mean 'you're welcome'. So when your family and friends thank you for making such a delicious and healthy dip just tell them, "Anoush".

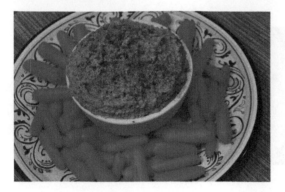

Here's what you need:

- 1 eggplant
- 3 Tablespoons olive oil
- juice from 1 lemon
- 1 Tablespoon balsamic vinegar
- 2 garlic cloves (or 2 cubes of Trader Joe's frozen minced garlic)
- 2 cups raw pecans
- 1/2 teaspoon sea salt
- dash of ground pepper

1. Preheat oven to 425 degrees F.
2. Wash eggplant and poke all over with a fork. Place on a foil-lined baking sheet and bake for 40 minutes.
3. Allow eggplant to cool. Remove the stem and peel away the skin. Place the eggplant insides in food processor.
4. Add the remaining ingredients and blend until smooth.
5. Serve with sliced veggies, or spread onto a sandwich.

Makes 12 servings

Nutritional Analysis: One serving equals: 176.8 calories, 17.8g fat, 66mg sodium, 6g carbohydrate, 20.5g fiber, and 2.3g protein

Sun-Dried Tomato & Basil Hummus

Sun-dried tomatoes and basil take this hummus to a whole new level of yumminess. You've gotta try it!

Homemade hummus always tastes better than store-bought hummus, and it is exceptionally easy to make. Can you throw a handful of ingredients into a food processor? Then you can make delicious homemade hummus!

Feel free to double the recipe — hummus keeps well and is a welcome addition to sandwiches, along side crackers or as a dip for fresh veggies.

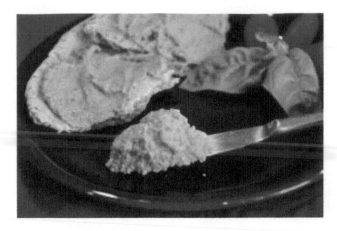

Here's what you need:

- 1 (15 oz) can garbanzo beans
- 2 Tablespoons tahini (feel free to leave this out if you're on a strict low-fat diet)
- 1 Tablespoon olive oil
- 1 Tablespoon lemon juice
- 1 Tablespoon water
- 2 garlic cloves, mashed
- 1/4 teaspoon salt
- 2 teaspoons soy sauce
- 4-6 sun-dried tomatoes
- 1/4 cup basil leaves

1. Throw all the ingredients into a food processor and combine until smooth. For a thinner consistency add water, 2 Tablespoons at a time.

Makes 12 servings

Nutritional Analysis: One serving equals: 72.8 calories, 2.8g fat, 100mg sodium, 8.5g carbohydrate, 2.2g fiber, and 3g protein

Roasted Red Pepper Spread

This spread is easy to make, tastes delicious and can be used as an appetizer spread on crackers or as a tasty topping for sandwich bread.

I recommend roasting your own peppers on a grill pan — simply heat the pan, throw the peppers on whole and place a lid directly on top of the peppers. Turn the peppers until each side is blackened, then place the peppers in a paper bag, close the top and let them sit for 10-15 minutes, this makes for easy peeling. Once they've cooled, peel off the skin and clean out the seeds.

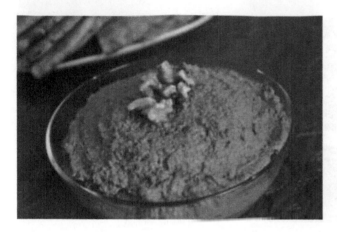

Here's what you need:

- 3 roasted red peppers
- 3 slices Ezekiel bread, toasted and processed in food processor into crumbs
- 1 cup toasted walnuts (place walnuts in toaster oven for a few minutes, watch closely to prevent burning!)
- 4 whole garlic cloves, peeled and mashed
- 1/2 teaspoon salt
- 1 Tablespoon lemon juice
- 2 teaspoons agave nectar
- 1 teaspoon cumin
- 1 teaspoon paprika

1. Throw all of the ingredients into a food processor and puree until it becomes smooth.

Makes 12 servings

Nutritional Analysis: One serving equals: 97.4 calories, 6.5g fat, 95.3mg sodium, 7.7g carbohydrate, 2.2g fiber, and 3g protein

Dressed Avocado

My mother-in-law introduced me to this method of dressing avocado. Since she has both an ever-producing lemon tree and a huge avocado tree, she makes it often. It is a delicious and speedy side dish!

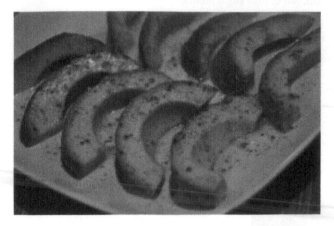

Here's what you need:

- Avocado, sliced
- Freshly squeezed lemon juice
- Dash of paprika
- Dash of garlic salt

1. Slice your avocado, generously drizzle it with lemon juice and then sprinkle with paprika and garlic salt. That's it!

Makes 2 servings

Nutritional Analysis: One serving equals: 147 calories, 13.4g fat, 69.7mg sodium, 8.3g carbohydrate, 6g fiber, and 1.8g protein

Nuts Spiced and Roasted

Nothing gets me into the holiday mood like the smell of spiced and roasted nuts. This recipe is super quick to make — literally 15 minutes. Put a bowl of these out when you have company over, take a bag of them with you for an on-the-go snack, or give it away as a healthy holiday gift, rather than sugar bombs.

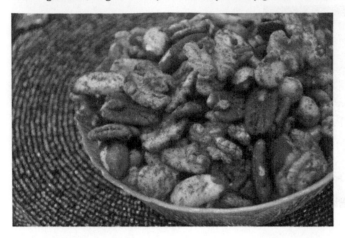

Here's what you need:

- 8 cups assorted nuts
- 2 Tablespoons organic butter
- 2 teaspoons vanilla extract
- 1/2 teaspoon almond extract
- 1 Tablespoon ground cumin
- 1 Tablespoon cinnamon
- dash of salt
- dash of nutmeg
- dash of red pepper

1. Use a large skillet to roast the nuts over medium heat. This will take about 5 minutes.
2. Meanwhile prepare a baking sheet by lining it with wax paper. Set aside.
3. Add the butter and once it melts coat all of the nuts evenly.
4. Add the vanilla and almond extracts and the spices. Mix well and continue to roast for a few minutes. Your kitchen will start to smell heavenly at this point!
5. Remove the nuts from heat and spread evenly over the prepared baking sheet. Allow to cool.

Makes 24 servings

Nutritional Analysis: One serving equals: 235.8 calories, 22.3g fat, 30mg sodium, 2.3g carbohydrate, 1.8g fiber, and 6.2g protein

Amazing Savory Cashews

These nuts are crazy good. Perfect for mid-day snacking or chopped and thrown onto a salad. Make plenty, because these disappear quickly.

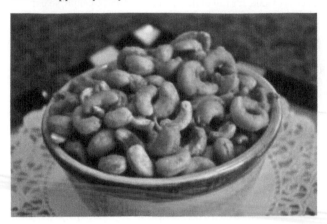

Here's what you need:

- 9 cups raw cashews
- 2 cups Nama Shoyu (unpasteurized soy sauce)
- 5 cups water
- 1/4 cup garlic powder
- 1/4 cup onion powder
- 1/4 cup lemon juice

1. Place the cashews in a large bowl. Pour the Nama Shoyu and water over the nuts — all nuts should be submerged. Allow to soak overnight.
2. Drain the nuts and mix in the remaining ingredients. Spread over dehydrator sheets and dry at 110 degrees until crunchy. (12-24 hrs)

Makes 30 servings

Nutritional Analysis: One serving equals: 244.3 calories, 16.8g fat, 958.7mg sodium, 13.7g carbohydrate, 8.7g fiber, and 7.3g protein

Cheesy Kale Chips

I love these chips because you get all the satisfaction of crunching on cheesy chips not only without guilt, but with the pleasure of knowing that you are getting all the benefits of kale. It's full of fiber, vitamin A and calcium, so eat up!

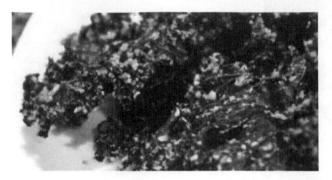

Here's what you need:

- 3 bunches organic, red kale, wash and trim the stems
- 1/4 cup cold pressed olive oil
- 2 cups nutritional yeast
- 1 cup Parma (or use 1 cup ground raw walnuts)
- fresh ground sea salt

1. Place the kale in a large mixing bowl. Coat with oil and then sprinkle with the remaining ingredients. Mix until fully coated.
2. Spread the kale over mesh dehydrator trays. Dehydrate at 115 degrees for 4 hours, or until desired crunchiness.

Makes 8 servings

Nutritional Analysis: One serving equals: 186.8 calories, 10.4g fat, 110.2mg sodium, 15.7g carbohydrate, 4.3g fiber, and 12.2g protein

Tasty Tuna Boats

Here's a nutritious meal that can be made in minutes. Red grapes, green apple and celery add a nice crunch to tender tuna and the avocado boat is fun for kids and adults alike.

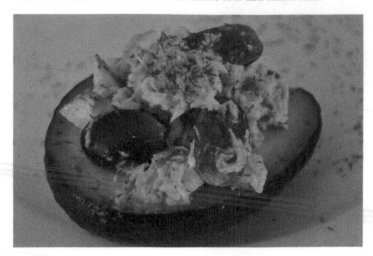

Here's what you need:

- 2 cans of wild caught albacore tuna, packed in water
- 2 celery stalks, finely chopped
- half of green apple, finely chopped
- 1/2 cup red grapes, halved
- 1/4 cup organic mayo
- 1 teaspoon dried dill weed, and more for garnish
- 3 Avocados, pitted and halved

1. Drain tuna, then flake into a medium bowl.
2. Add the remaining ingredients, except avocado, and mix until well combined.
3. Serve by placing a scoop of tuna into each avocado half. Sprinkle with dill weed.

Makes 6 servings

Nutritional Analysis: One serving equals: 268.3 calories, 22.3g fat, 147.3mg sodium, 13.3g carbohydrate, 7.5g fiber, and 11.3g protein

Veggie Hand Rolls

Living in southern California, where we have a sushi joint on every corner, I've come to love this very veggie version of a hand roll. I mean, who really said that sushi has to have meat in it?

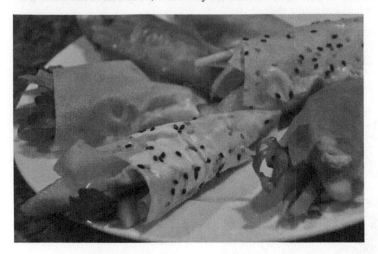

Here's what you need:

- 5 soy wrappers, cut in half
- 1/4 cup toffuti cream cheese
- 1/2 cucumber, cut into matchsticks
- 3 carrots, cut into matchsticks
- 1/2 red bell pepper, cut into matchsticks
- 1/2 mango, thinly sliced
- 1/2 cup baby arugula
- 1/4 cup pickled ginger
- 1 avocado, sliced and seasoned
- soy sauce for dipping

1. Prepare all of the veggies and arrange on a large cutting board.
2. Assemble each hand roll by placing a couple of each veggie in the center of a soy wrapper. Smear a touch of tofutti on one edge of the wrapper, then roll and press down the edge to seal.
3. Serve with soy sauce.

Makes 5 servings

Nutritional Analysis: One serving equals: 164.8 calories, 8.8g fat, 132.4mg sodium, 18.9g carbohydrate, 4.1g fiber, and 1.2g protein

Fun Fruit Skewers

Here's a fun idea for serving fruit at a party.

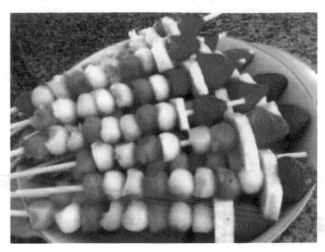

Here's what you need:

- Wooden skewers (I found these thick ones in the cake decorating section at WalMart — these don't have pointed ends)
- 1 small watermelon
- 1 small cantaloupe
- 1 small honeydew
- 1 pineapple
- 20 large strawberries

1. Slice the melons in half and use a melon baller to create red, orange and green melon balls.
2. Twist the top off the pineapple, slice the skin off and cut out the tough core. Slice 20 triangular pieces, carefully cut a small X in the center of each piece.
3. Use a slightly damp paper towel to wipe down the strawberries (this will prevent them from getting soggy).
4. To assemble: slide 8 melon balls in alternating colors onto each skewer, top with a slice of pineapple and a strawberry.

Makes 20 servings

Nutritional Analysis: One serving equals: 73.8 calories, .3g fat, 14mg sodium, 18.3g carbohydrate, 1.6g fiber, and 1.3g protein

Strawberry MicroGreen Salad

This strawberry microgreen salad is perfect– it's sweet, has small easy-to-chew microgreens, and is peppered with sliced strawberries and candied walnuts.

If you're in a hurry you can purchase pre-made strawberry salad dressing and packaged candied walnuts rather than making them.

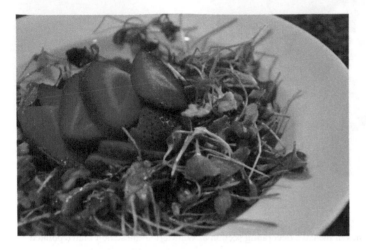

Here's what you need:

- 3 cups organic microgreens
- 1 cup sliced strawberry
- strawberry dressing (6 strawberries, 1 Tablespoon balsamic vinegar, 1 teaspoon agave nectar, 2 tablespoons olive oil, dash of salt and pepper — blended)
- 1/4 cup chopped candied walnuts

1. Toss the microgreens with strawberries and dressing. Sprinkle with walnuts.

Makes 2 servings

Nutritional Analysis: One serving equals: 200.5 calories, 13.3g fat, 196mg sodium, 19.2g carbohydrate, 4.7g fiber, and 3.8g protein

Fruity Fennel Salad

I'll admit that before trying this recipe I didn't even know what fennel bulb was–what a revelation! This white bulb packs amazing flavor, reminiscent to black licorice (in a good way).

Pomegranate seeds add beautiful color while the orange pieces contribute a hint of tangy citrus and pecan pieces round it out with a satisfying, buttery crunch.

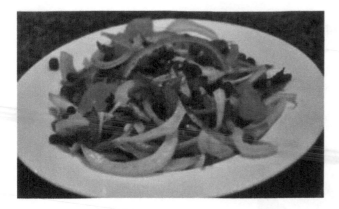

Here's what you need:

- 1 Fennel bulb, sliced (it's that white bulb-looking thing with the green stalks in the produce section)
- 1/2 red onion, sliced
- 1 orange peeled, cut into bite-sized chunks
- 1/3 cup pecan pieces, toasted
- 1/2 cup pomegranate seeds
- 2 garlic cloves, minced
- 1/4 cup fresh squeezed orange juice
- 1/4 cup rice vinegar
- 1 teaspoon agave nectar
- handful of mint leaves, chopped

1. In a medium bowl combine fennel, onion, orange pieces, pecan pieces and pomegranate.
2. In a small bowl whisk together garlic, orange juice, rice vinegar, agave nectar and mint leaves.
3. Pour the dressing over the salad and toss until well combined.

Tip: Trader Joe's sells fresh pomegranate seeds, so you can save yourself from the hassle of cutting and seeding it yourself (messy!)

Makes 2 servings

Nutritional Analysis: One serving equals: 308.5 calories, 14.9g fat, 62mg sodium, 41.8g carbohydrate, 8.7g fiber, and 6g protein

Real Healthy Tomato Salad

Oh the bounty of summer!

Garden fresh heirloom and cherry tomatoes come in unique colors and flavors — all ripe for the pickin' and all filled with anti-oxidant rich Lycopene.

This salad is fresh, flavorful and so simple to throw together.

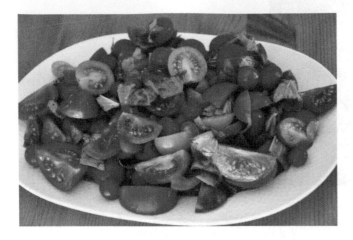

Here's what you need for 5 servings:

- 1.5 lbs assorted fresh tomatoes
- 1 cup fresh basil leaves
- 2 Tablespoons balsamic vinegar
- 1 Tablespoon olive oil
- 1 clove garlic
- dash of cracked pepper
- 1 packet Stevia
- juice from 1/2 a lemon

1. Wash the tomatoes and slice the larger ones into halves or quarters. Place in a medium bowl.
2. Wash the basil leaves, pat dry. Set 10 leaves aside. Chop the remaining leaves roughly and add to the bowl.
3. Combine the 10 basil leaves, balsamic vinegar, olive oil, garlic, pepper, stevia and lemon juice in a high speed blender. Blend on high until fully combined.
4. Pour the dressing over the tomato mixture. Chill for one hour in refrigerator. Drain off dressing and serve.

Makes 5 Servings

Nutritional Analysis: One serving equals: 47 calories, 3g fat, 6mg sodium, 4 carbohydrate, 1g fiber, and 1g protein.

Gourmet Spring Salad

This salad is bursting with Spring flavors. Curly endive and dandelion greens combine with fresh asparagus, cherry tomatoes, red bell pepper, red onion and tender hard boiled eggs in a delicious oil-free dressing.

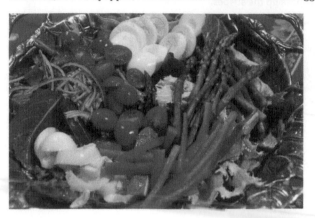

Here's what you need:

- 4 organic, omega-3 eggs
- 1 bunch asparagus, ends trimmed
- 1 cup curly endive
- 1 cup dandelion greens
- 1/2 cup cherry tomatoes, halved
- 1/8 cup red onion, thinly sliced
- 1/2 red bell pepper, thinly sliced into matchsticks
- 2 Tablespoons agave nectar
- 2 Tablespoons lime juice
- 1 garlic clove, minced
- 2 teaspoons Dijon mustard
- 1 Tablespoon raspberry vinegar

1. Place the eggs in a pan of water, bring to a simmer for 6 minutes. Remove from heat. Crack the eggs all over, then place in a pan of cold water for one minute. Remove from water, peel, and slice. Set aside.
2. Bring a medium pot of salted water to boil. Add the asparagus and cook for 4 minutes. Rinse in cold water then set aside.
3. In a large salad bowl combine the endive, dandelion greens, tomato, onion and pepper.
4. In a small bowl combine the agave, lime juice, garlic, dijon and vinegar. Mix well.
5. Coat the salad with the dressing. Top with asparagus and sliced egg.

Makes 4 servings

Nutritional Analysis: One serving equals: 137.5 calories, 5.7g fat, 270mg sodium, 11.4g carbohydrate, 3.3g fiber, and 10.6g protein

World's Best Cobb Salad

Everyone loves this massive Cobb salad. By arranging the toppings in stripes you'll create a stunning presentation. Once it's time to eat, let your guests know that it OK to mess up the stripes.

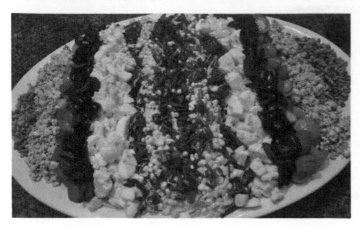

Here's what you need:

- 2 bags of Butter Lettuce (or 2 heads of butter lettuce, chopped)
- 6 hard boiled eggs
- 1 cup fresh corn kernels
- 1 cup kalamata olives, halved
- 1 cup cherry tomatoes, halved
- 1 cup blue cheese crumbles
- 1/2 cup pine nuts, toasted
- 1 cup shredded purple cabbage
- 1/4 cup chives, chopped
- 1 cup cooked turkey bacon, chopped
- Your choice of dressing

1. Spread the butter lettuce over a large platter.
2. Start by creating a line of turkey bacon down the center of the lettuce, then create identical lines of toppings on either side of the bacon.
3. Serve with dressing on the side.

Makes 12 servings

Nutritional Analysis (without dressing): One serving equals: 165 calories, 11.2g fat, 379.6mg sodium, 7.6g carbohydrate, 2g fiber, and 9.3g protein

Roasted Veggie Salad with Couscous

When is a salad not just a salad? When it has gorgeous presentation. This recipe not only looks beautiful, it tastes amazing and works as a filling main dish. I highly recommend using a glass bowl so that each scrumptious layer will be appreciated.

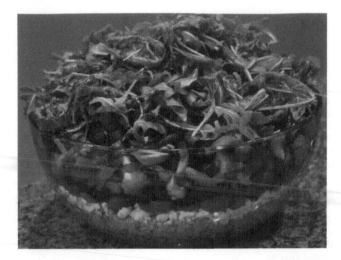

Here's what you need:

For the Dressing:

- 1 lemon, juiced
- 1 Tablespoon tomato paste
- 2 teaspoons ground coriander seed
- 2 teaspoons ground cumin
- dash of salt and pepper
- 1/2 cup olive oil
- 1/2 cup minced fresh parsley

For the Veggies:

- 1/4 cup olive oil
- 4 garlic cloves, minced
- 2 medium eggplants, cut into small cubes
- 2 green zucchini, halved and sliced
- 2 yellow zucchini, halved and sliced
- 1 small bunch carrots, sliced
- 1 red, 1 orange and 1 yellow bell peppers, seeded and cut into strips
- 1 large red onion, cut into large half-moons
- 1 cup pearl onions, halved
- dash of salt and pepper

For the Couscous:

- 1 Tablespoon olive oil
- dash of salt
- 1 cube veggie bouillon
- 5 oz package whole wheat couscous

For the Salad:

- 1 1/2 cups crumbled goat cheese
- 1 cup cherry tomatoes, halved
- 1/2 cup kalamta olives, pitted and halved
- 5oz baby arugula
- 2 Tablespoons balsamic vinegar

1. Make the dressing: In a small bowl whisk the lemon juice, tomato paste, coriander and cumin. Add the oil and parsley and season with salt and pepper. Set aside.
2. Make the veggies: Preheat oven to 375 degrees F, and position a rack at the center and one in the top third of the oven. Oil 2 large rimmed cookie sheets. Mix all the prepared veggies in a bowl, toss with the olive oil and minced garlic. Season with salt and pepper. Spread the veggies out over the two prepared sheets. Place in preheated oven for 20 minutes, then mix the veggies and switch the pan positions. Roast for an additional 20 minutes or until all the veggies are tender.
3. Make the Couscous: Bring 2 cups of water to a boil, add the oil, salt and bouillon. Add the couscous, stir, cover tightly and remove from heat. Allow to sit for 5 minutes, then fluff the couscous with a fork.
4. Assemble the salad: Use a large glass bowl to layer the ingredients in an artful way. Spread the couscous on the bottom of the bowl, drizzle with a few tablespoons of dressing. Top with the goat cheese, cherry tomatoes and olives. Add the roasted veggies and drizzle with more of the dressing. In a separate bowl, mix the arugula with balsamic vinegar then place on the top of the roasted veggies.

Makes 20 servings

Nutritional Analysis: One serving equals: 211 calories, 13.6g fat, 271.3mg sodium, 18.8g carbohydrate, 4.3g fiber, and 5.7g protein

Beverly Hills Chopped Salad

It seems to me that every restaurant in Beverly Hills features a chopped salad as their most popular dish. This recipe is part Villa Blanca, part The Ivy and is fully delicious! The dressing is my absolute favorite.

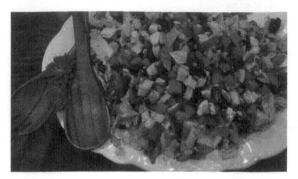

Here's what you need:

- 1 bunch asparagus, chopped
- 4 large carrots, chopped
- 5 green onions, chopped
- 1 green zucchini
- 1 yellow zucchini
- 1 teaspoon olive oil
- dash of salt and pepper
- 1 avocado, chopped
- 2 heads of romaine lettuce, chopped
- 1/2 cup cherry tomatoes, chopped
- 1/4 cup kalamata olives, chopped
- 1/4 cup pine nuts, toasted

For the dressing:

- 1/8 cup olive oil
- 2 Tablespoons lime juice
- 2 Tablespoons agave nectar
- 1 clove garlic, minced (or better yet use one frozen garlic cube from Trader Joes)
- 1 teaspoon champagne mustard

1. Preheat oven to 425 degrees F. Place the asparagus, carrot, onion and zucchinis in a large bowl, mix well with the olive oil and salt and pepper. Place on a baking sheet and roast for 20 minutes, stirring after the first 10 minutes.
2. Meanwhile place the remaining salad ingredients into a large bowl. In a small bowl combine all of the dressing ingredients and whisk with a fork.
3. Once the veggies are roasted, mix into the salad bowl and toss with the dressing.

Makes 4-6 servings

Nutritional Analysis: One serving equals: 236.3 calories, 14.5g fat, 147.6mg sodium, 25.6g carbohydrate, 8.1g fiber, and 6.1g protein

Manly Man Salad

Let's be honest — manly men don't typically love salads.

They'd rather sit down to a nice big juicy piece of steak than a dainty plate of greens.

This salad is anything but dainty, with bacon, eggs and hearty spinach. It will please even the manliest man in your life

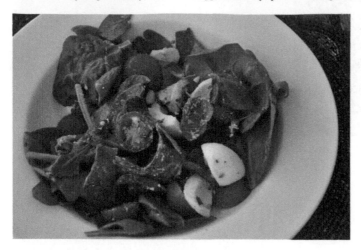

Here's what you need for 4 servings:

- 6 cups organic baby spinach
- 4 hard boiled eggs, chopped
- 6 pieces bacon, crumbled
- 1 cup cherry tomatoes, halved
- 1 teaspoon olive oil
- Juice from one lime
- dash of pepper

1. Combine the spinach, eggs, bacon and tomatoes in a large bowl.
2. In a small bowl whisk the olive oil, lime juice and pepper.
3. Pour the dressing over the salad, mix and serve.

4 Servings

Nutritional Analysis: One serving equals: 170 calories, 10g fat, 337mg sodium, 5g carbohydrate, 2g fiber, and 13g protein

Real Simple Fruit Salad

Fruit salad is a staple of summer.

Juicy melons, sweet berries and crisp apples eaten from a paper plate while the sunshine warms your head.

When the fruit is sweet and at its peak, there's no need for extra sweeteners.

A squeeze of fresh lime, a sprinkle of chopped mint and you're good to go.

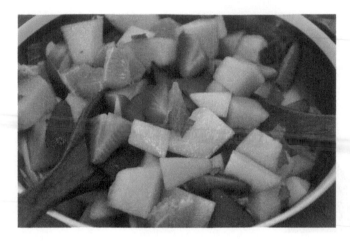

Here's what you need:

- 1 honeydew melon, chopped
- 2 crisp apples, chopped
- 1 orange, peeled and chopped
- 1 cup sliced strawberries
- 15 mint leaves, minced
- 2 Tablespoons fresh lime juice

1. Combine the fruit in a large bowl.
2. In a small cup combine the mint and lime.
3. Drizzle lime mixture over the fruit and toss well.

Makes 6 servings

Nutritional Analysis: One serving equals: 117 calories, 0.2g fat, 33.4mg sodium, 31g carbohydrate, 3.6g fiber, and 1.8g protein.

Quinoa Minty Fruit Salad

Quinoa is quite the superfood.

Often mistaken for a grain, quinoa is actually a protein-packed seed. It's gluten free (yay!) and is a complete protein, containing all 9 essential amino acids. It is also filled with magnesium and fiber, as if the other benefits weren't enough to convince us.

The one drawback to this amazing food is the carbohydrate volume. While it is lower than rice or other traditional grains, it is high enough that you'll want to limit the amount you eat.

Most quinoa recipes are savory, so this minty, fruity salad is a refreshing twist on the nutritious-packed superfood.

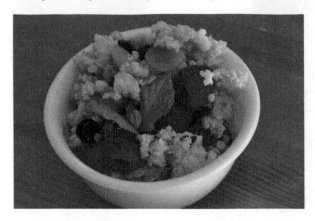

Here's what you need for 6 servings:

- 3/4 cup plain greek yogurt
- 2 Tablespoons lime juice, divided
- 1-15 fresh mint leaves, minced
- 2 cups cooked quinoa
- dash of salt and pepper
- 1 cup blueberries
- 1 cup green grapes, halved
- 1/2 cup raspberries
- 1 Tablespoon agave nectar

1. In a small bowl combine the yogurt, 1 tablespoon lime juice and the mint. Pour over the cooked quinoa and mix well. Season with salt and pepper.
2. In another bowl combine the fruit, agave nectar and remaining lime juice.
3. Cover and refrigerate each bowl for 2 hours, to allow the flavors to emerge, then combine the fruit with the quinoa and serve.

Makes 6 Servings

Nutritional Analysis: One serving equals: 139 calories, 1g fat, 114mg sodium, 27g carbohydrate, 3g fiber, and 6g protein.

Real Healthy Egg Salad

When egg salad is done right it is delicious, creamy and satisfying. When egg salad is done wrong it is tasteless, mushy and heavy.

This Real Healthy Egg Salad is made with nonfat Greek yogurt, fresh celery and onion greens. It is perfect on a bed of lettuce, wrapped in romaine lettuce leaves or in a sprouted grain tortilla. This is egg salad done right.

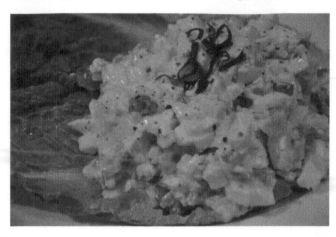

Here's what you need:

- 8 organic, free range eggs
- 4 celery stalks, chopped
- 2 Tablespoons onion greens, chopped
- 1/4 cup non fat Greek yogurt
- 2 teaspoons champagne mustard
- 1 teaspoon fresh squeezed lemon
- dash of salt and pepper

1. To boil the perfect egg: place eggs in a large pot and cover with cold water by half an inch. Heat the water to a boil, turn off the heat and cover the pot. Wait exactly 7 minutes, and then place the eggs in a bowl of ice water for 3 minutes.
2. Peel and chop hard boiled eggs. Place in a large bowl. Add celery, onion greens, yogurt, mustard, lemon, salt and pepper. Mix well.
3. Chill and then serve.

Makes 4 servings

Nutritional Analysis: One serving equals: 174 calories, 10.7g fat, 229.2mg sodium, 3.4g carbohydrate, .7g fiber, and 14.5g protein

Creamy Tuna Salad with Apple and Cabbage

This recipe turned out impossibly delicious and creamy, thanks to fat-free Greek yogurt. Shredded apple and green cabbage compliment the creaminess with a delicate crunch.

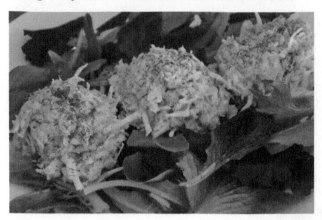

Here's what you need for 4 servings:

- 2 (5oz) cans wild albacore tuna, packed in water
- 1 cup fat-free Greek yogurt
- 2 Tablespoons champagne mustard
- 1 teaspoon dried dill weed, plus more for garnish
- dash of freshly ground pepper
- 1 green apple, shredded
- 2 cups green cabbage, shredded
- 4 cups organic mixed greens

1. Drain the tuna and flake in a medium bowl. Add the yogurt, mustard, dill and pepper. Mix until creamy and well combined.
2. Add the shredded apple and cabbage. Mix well.
3. Arrange mixed greens on plates, then use an ice cream scooper to place the tuna mixture. Sprinkle with dill weed.

Makes 4 servings

Nutritional Analysis: One serving equals: 122.5 calories, 0.4g fat, 264.3mg sodium, 13g carbohydrate, 2.8g fiber, and 16.8g protein

Chicken Salad with Mango Chutney

This mango chutney covered chicken salad is perfect for a summer dinner — no oven required!

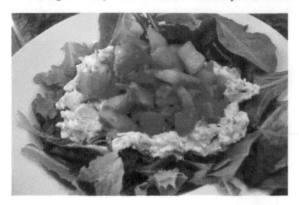

Here's what you need for 5 servings:

- 1 teaspoon olive oil
- 2 cloves garlic, minced
- 1 inch ginger root, minced
- 1 small red onion, chopped
- 1 small red bell pepper, chopped
- 2 ripe mangoes, chopped
- Juice from 2 limes
- 1 Tablespoon curry powder
- 1 teaspoon ground cinnamon
- Dash of nutmeg
- Dash of red pepper flakes
- 1 ½ cups non-fat, plain Greek yogurt
- 1 Tablespoon Dijon mustard
- Dash of salt and pepper
- 3 cups cooked chicken breast, chopped
- 4 cups salad greens

1. In a large skillet, heat oil over medium heat. Add garlic and ginger root and sauté for a minute.
2. Add the onion and bell peppers and sauté for a few minutes.
3. Add the mango and spices. Continue to sauté for another 5 minutes, until everything has softened.
4. Turn the heat down to low, cover and simmer for another 10 minutes. Remove from heat. Chill for 20 minutes in the refrigerator.
5. Combine the yogurt, mustard, salt and pepper together in a small bowl. Place the chopped chicken in a medium sized bowl and mix in the yogurt blend.
6. Prepare each plate with a pile of greens topped with a scoop of chicken and a spoonful of chutney.

Makes 4 servings

Nutritional Analysis: One serving equals: 286 calories, 6 fat, 185mg sodium, 22g carbohydrates, 3g fiber, and 35g protein.

Tropical Chopped Chicken Salad

This salad was inspired by the recent burst of sun we've been enjoying — making me long for a tropical get-away with white sand beaches and juicy mangoes. Oh how I love mangoes.

The mango dressing I found turned out to be amazing as both the marinade and the dressing!

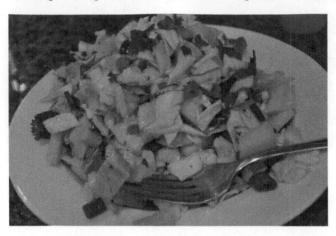

Here's what you need:

- 4 skinless chicken breast, organic and vegetarian fed
- Bolthouse Farms Tropical Mango Olive Oil Vinegrette
- 1 head cabbage, chopped
- 1 red bell pepper, chopped
- 1 mango, chopped
- ½ cup pineapple, chopped
- 1 bunch cilantro, chopped
- 1/3 cup green onions, chopped

1. Rinse the chicken breasts and place in a large ziplock bag. Pour in enough of the Mango Vinegrette to fully cover the chicken. Place in the fridge for at least 4 hours.
2. Preheat oven to 350 degrees F and grease a pan with coconut oil.
3. Bake the marinated chicken breasts for 30 minutes until cooked through, then turn on the broiler for 3-5 minutes until deeply golden. Chop and set aside.
4. In a large bowl combine all of the remaining ingredients along with the chopped chicken. Drizzle a little of the mango vinegrette and mix well.

Makes 5 servings

Nutritional Analysis: One serving equals: 240.6 calories, 3.6g fat, 285.8mg sodium, 23.5g carbohydrate, 5.9g fiber, and 28.6g protein

Pesto Spaghetti Squash Salad

Squash abounds this time of year. The produce section has piles of them, and you see recipes for baked squash, creamed squash, even for squash pies. My inspiration for this salad was to do something new with squash — to create something crisp and refreshing. With very few ingredients, this salad has powerful flavor. You'll love how the distinct flavor of fennel mingles with fresh pesto.

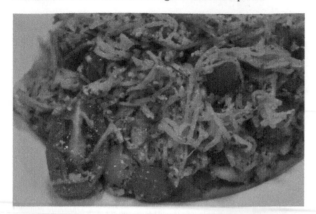

Here's what you need:

- 1 spaghetti squash
- 2-3 cup basil leaves
- 1/2 cup pine nuts
- 3 cloves garlic (or 3 frozen minced cubes from Trader Joes)
- 1/4 cup olive oil
- 1 Tablespoon fresh lemon juice
- dash of salt
- 2 fennel bulbs
- 2 lbs organic cherry tomatoes

1. Cut the spaghetti squash in half, and scoop out the seeds. Run water over the insides of the squash. Microwave each half, separately, for 5 minutes. Use an dishtowel to remove from microwave — it will be HOT! Set aside and allow to cool, then place in the fridge for at least 15 minutes.
2. In a food processor, combine the basil leaves, pine nuts, and garlic. Combine while you drizzle in the olive oil. Add the lemon juice and a dash of salt. Once a paste forms, remove from food processor.
3. Scoop the cooled spaghetti squash from its skin, and place into a large bowl. Use a knife to cut up the large bunches of squash. Thinly slice the fennel bulb into 1 inch segments and add to the bowl. Mix in the pesto until everything is well coated.
4. Cut larger cherry tomatoes in half, and leave smaller ones intact. Add all the tomatoes to the bowl and mix well. Taste the salad, and use another dash of salt if needed.

Makes 8 servings

Nutritional Analysis: One serving equals: 172.5 calories, 12.6g fat, 78.3mg sodium, 14.4g carbohydrate, 4.4g fiber, and 3.4g protein

Amazing Cauliflower Rice

Not many people realize that cauliflower is a great source of vitamin C. And that is just a bonus when it comes to this savory recipe. By decreasing (or eliminating) the amount of grains that you include in your diet, you will quickly start to lose weight and lean out. This recipe is great for those days when you want to eat rice, but still want to stick to your diet.

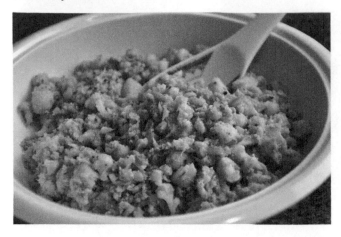

Here's what you need:

- 1 red onion, minced
- 3 garlic cloves, minced (buy the frozen garlic trays at Trader Joes, then simply pop 3 cubes out)
- 1 Tablespoon basil, diced (buy the frozen basil trays at Trader Joes, then simply pop 4 cubes out)
- 1 head of organic cauliflower, stem removed.
- 2 eggs
- 3 Tablespoon coconut flour
- 2 teaspoon freshly ground sea salt
- 4 Tablespoons coconut oil

1. Cut cauliflower into small pieces with stems removed. Steam it until soft.
2. In a large bowl combine onions, garlic, basil, cauliflower, eggs, coconut flour, salt and pepper. Mash it down to the consistency of rice.
3. Heat coconut oil in large skillet over medium heat. Add the cauliflower mixture and saute for 10-15 minutes, until tender.

Makes 6 servings

Nutritional Analysis: One serving equals: 160.1 calories, 11.6g fat, 574mg sodium, 9.2g carbohydrate, 4g fiber, and 5g protein

Quinoa with Basil and Almonds

Quinoa is always a great addition to a nutritious meal. I consider it my protein-rich go-to grain (even though it is technically a seed). This recipe is quick and is a great way to use fresh-from-the-garden basil.

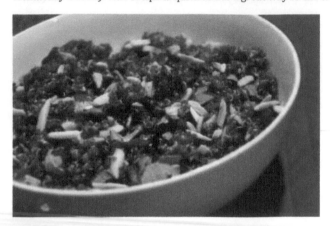

Here's what you need:

- 1 cup quinoa
- dash of sea salt
- 1/2 cup slivered almonds
- 1/2 cup fresh basil leaves, chopped

1. In a saucepan combine the quinoa with 2 cups of water and the salt. Bring to a boil then reduce to a simmer and cover for 20 mins.
2. Heat the slivered almonds in a dry skillet over medium heat. Toast until golden brown.
3. Transfer the cooked quinoa to a serving bowl and mix in the almonds and basil.

Makes 2 servings

Nutritional Analysis: One serving equals: 267 calories, 15g fat, 132mg sodium, 25.8g carbohydrate, 5.9g fiber, and 9.9g protein

Roasted Brussels Sprouts & Caramelized Green Apples

This recipe combines roasted Brussels Sprouts with tender green apples for a truly wonderful flavor. If you're not sure how you feel about Brussels Sprouts, this is a great recipe to try — but don't be surprised if you get hooked!

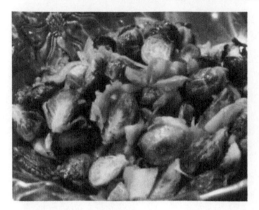

Here's what you need:

- 40 Brussels Sprouts (about 1.5 lbs) trimmed and halved
- 1 Tablespoon olive oil
- Dash of salt and pepper
- 1 Tablespoon nonhydrogenated vegan butter (EarthBalance)
- 1 large yellow onion, thinly sliced
- 4 green apples, thinly sliced
- 1 teaspoon agave nectar

1. Preheat oven to 425 degrees. In a large mixing bowl combine Brussels sprouts, olive oil, salt and pepper. Spread over a baking sheet and place in the oven for 20 to 40 minutes. Mix the sprouts every 10 minutes to ensure even roasting. You'll know the sprouts are done when they turn a dark brown and are tender.
2. Meanwhile in a large skillet, melt the Earth Balance over low-medium heat. Add the onions, apples and agave nectar. Cook, stirring occasionally for about 30 minutes, until the onions and apples are golden brown and caramelized.
3. Combine the Brussels sprouts and the apple mixture in a large bowl. Enjoy!

Makes 4 servings

Nutritional Analysis: One serving equals: 236.5 calories, 13g fat, 138mg sodium, 43.7g carbohydrate, 12.9g fiber, and 7g protein

Garlicky Asparagus

Here's an awesome asparagus recipe. It's simple and quick and tastes great.

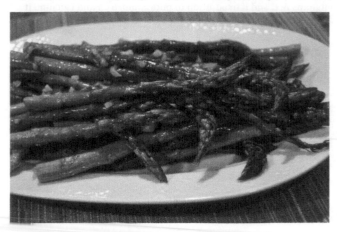

Here's what you need:

- 1 bunch asparagus
- 2 teaspoons olive oil
- 1 ½ Tablespoons garlic, minced
- dash of salt and pepper
- 2 teaspoons lemon juice

1. Preheat oven to 425 degrees F. Cut off the tough ends of the asparagus.
2. In a casserole dish, combine the asparagus, oil, garlic, salt and pepper. Bake for 15-20 minutes, until tender.
3. Remove from oven and mix in the lemon juice. Serve and enjoy!

Makes 4 servings

Nutritional Analysis: One serving equals: 50 calories, 2.5g fat, 66.3mg sodium, 6.2g carbohydrate, 2.9g fiber, and 3g protein

Sauteed Broccoli Rabe

Here's a quick way to dress up broccoli rabe. Broccoli rabe is a non-heading type of broccoli with long thin leafy stalks, topped with small florets. It's packed with vitamins A, C and K in addition to potassium, iron and calcium. It also contains phytochemicals that fight cancer and improve your overall health.

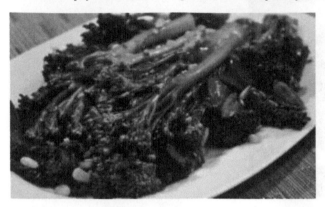

Here's what you need:

- 3 Tablespoons pine nuts, toasted
- 2 bunches broccoli rabe, stems trimmed
- 1 Tablespoon olive oil
- 3 garlic cloves, minced
- 1/4 cup kalamata olives, halved
- dash of freshly ground sea salt
- Juice from 1 small lemon

1. Place a steamer basket over a 3 quart pot, filled with water up to the bottom of the basket. Bring the water to a boil, add the broccoli, cover and steam for 3 minutes. Immediately drop the broccoli into a bowl of ice water. After a few minutes drain the broccoli and set aside.
2. In a large skillet warm the olive oil over medium heat. Add the garlic and saute until golden. Add the broccoli, olives and salt. Saute for another 5 minutes until tender. Remove from heat, place in serving dish, sprinkle with pine nuts and toss with lemon juice.

Makes 4 servings

Nutritional Analysis: One serving equals: 99 calories, 8.6g fat, 158.7mg sodium, 5.1g carbohydrate, 1.8g fiber, and 3g protein

Favorite Green Beans

Green beans are low in calories and packed with vitamins. This dish is quick to whip together and the flavors are deliciously tangy.

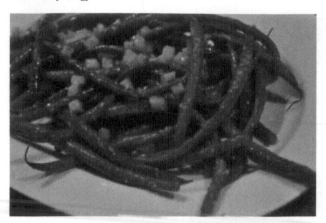

Here's what you need:

- 8oz green beans
- 2 teaspoons olive oil
- 1 Tablespoon dijon mustard
- 2 teaspoons brown rice vinegar
- 3 Tablespoons diced yellow onion
- dash of salt and pepper

1. Steam the green beans until soft, yet still with a slight crunch.
2. In a medium bowl whisk together the remaining ingredients. Add the green beans and toss together.
3. Transfer beans to serving dish and enjoy.

Makes 4 servings

Nutritional Analysis: One serving equals: 77 calories, 7g fat, 154.2mg sodium, 2.6g carbohydrate, 1g fiber, and 0.6g protein

Tender Summer Squash

Here's another option when it comes to summer squash. This year my garden has been taken over by zucchini and yellow squash, so this recipe has come in handy!

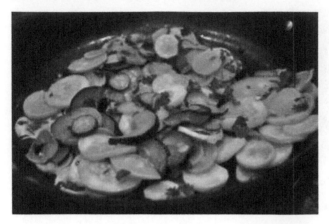

Here's what you need:

- 2 lbs summer squash
- 1 Tablespoon olive oil
- 3 cloves garlic, chopped
- 1/2 cup water
- freshly ground sea salt and pepper
- 1/3 cup parsley, chopped
- handful of basil leaves, torn

1. Slice the squash into slices, about 1/4 inch thick
2. Heat the oil in a large skillet. Add the garlic. When the garlic is golden, add the squash and cook over med-low heat, flipping every 5 minutes for about 20 minutes.
3. Add the water and continue to cook until none remains. Season with the salt and pepper and sprinkle the herbs on top.

Makes 4 servings

Nutritional Analysis: One serving equals: 54 calories, 3.8g fat, 65.3mg sodium, 4.8g carbohydrate, 1.7g fiber, and 1.8g protein

Pickled Beets

This salad is delicious, with the added bonus that the beets will keep for much longer after you've 'pickled' them.

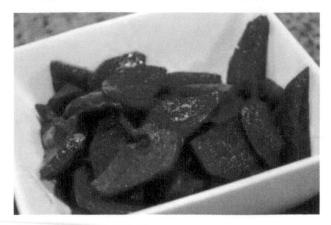

Here's what you need:

- 4 beets, peeled, sliced in half and cut into 1/8 inch slices
- 1/3 cup apple cider vinegar
- 1 Tablespoon agave nectar
- 1 teaspoon olive oil
- 1 teaspoon balsamic vinegar

1. Bring 1 cup of water to boil in a saucepan over medium heat. Add the beets and cover, boiling for 8 minutes. Remove from heat, drain the water and return to the pan.
2. Whisk together the apple cider vinegar, agave nectar, olive oil and balsamic vinegar in small bowl.
3. Return the beets to medium heat, add the vinegar mixture and simmer for 5 minutes. Cool before placing in airtight container in the fridge.

Makes 4 servings

Nutritional Analysis: One serving equals: 69.5 calories, 1.3g fat, 64mg sodium, 14.5g carbohydrate, 2.3g fiber, and 1.3g protein

Turkey & Veggie Comfort Stew

There's nothing better than a warm bowl of comforting stew — especially when it's filled with nutritious ingredients like veggies and lean ground turkey.

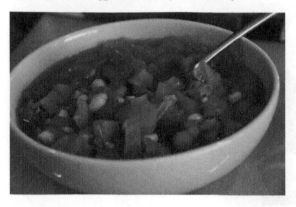

Here's what you need:

- 2 teaspoons olive oil
- 2 garlic cloves, minced (or save time with frozen minced garlic cubes from Trader Joes)
- 1 bunch of carrots, chopped
- 2 onions, chopped
- 1 bunch of celery
- 1 fennel bulb
- 1.3 lbs lean ground turkey
- 4 cups veggie broth
- 1 (14.5oz) can stewed tomatoes
- 1 (15oz) can white kidney beans
- 4 ears of corn, kernels sliced off cobb
- 3 Tablespoons tomato paste
- 2 teaspoons dried basil
- dash of salt and freshly ground pepper

1. In a large skillet heat the olive oil. Add garlic.
2. Add chopped carrots, cover for 5 minutes.
3. Add onions, celery and fennel. Saute until soft.
4. In another skillet cook the ground turkey over medium heat until fully cooked, stirring often. Drain off excess fat.
5. Transfer the veggies to large soup pot and add the remaining ingredients, and the cooked turkey. Cover and cook over low heat for 40 minutes. Add extra water as desired.

Makes 8 servings

Nutritional Analysis: One serving equals: 274.1 calories, 6.3g fat, 480.2mg sodium, 34g carbohydrate, 10.5g fiber, and 21.5g protein

Okra & Carrot Stew

Okra is one of my all time favorite comfort foods. There's something delicious about biting into the tender okra skin and then having the seeds pop in your mouth. This stew is incredibly simple and quick to make — perfect for a cold and gloomy day.

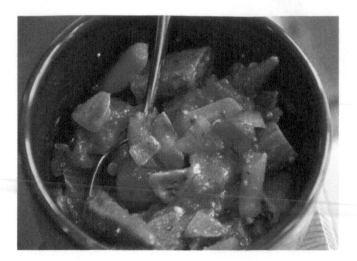

Here's what you need:

- 1 Tablespoon olive oil
- 4 cloves garlic, minced (or save time and use 4 cubes of frozen minced garlic from Trader Joe's)
- 1 cup baby carrots, sliced lengthwise and crosswise
- 1 large sweet onion, chopped
- 1 pound fresh okra
- 1 (28oz) can whole tomatoes
- 1 quart veggie broth (32oz)
- 1/2 teaspoon freshly ground peppercorns
- 1/4 teaspoon sea salt
- 1/2 teaspoon dried oregano
- 1/2 teaspoon ground cumin
- 1 teaspoon dried thyme

1. In a very large skillet, or medium pot, heat olive oil. Add garlic, carrots and onion. Cover and cook, stirring occasionally, for 5 minutes.
2. Meanwhile, trim the ends from Okra and cut in half crosswise.
3. Add okra, tomatoes, broth and spices to skillet. Gently break tomatoes apart with spoon. Mix and allow to cook, uncovered, on medium heat for 20-25 minutes, until okra is tender.

Makes 4 servings

Nutritional Analysis: One serving equals: 118 calories, 3.7g fat, 587.7mg sodium, 19.4g carbohydrate, 6g fiber, and 5.4g protein

Quinoa Harvest Stew

This simple stew combines fresh autumn vegetables with protein rich quinoa. I love making a huge pot of stew and then eating it for a few days in a row.

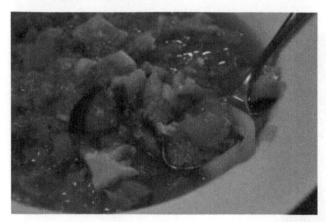

Here's what you need:

- 10 cups filtered water
- 1/4 cup soy sauce (I use Nama Shoyu – raw unpasteurized soy sauce)
- 1 cup uncooked quinoa
- 4 small potatoes, peeled and chopped
- 1 leek, chopped
- 4 garlic cloves, minced
- 2 zucchini, chopped
- 1 small head green cabbage, sliced
- 4-6 medium sized tomatoes
- 4-6 small carrots
- dash of freshly ground salt and pepper
- 2 Tablespoons dried parsley
- 2 teaspoons oregano

1. Place the water and soy sauce in a large soup pot over medium heat. Add the uncooked quinoa.
2. Allow the quinoa to simmer as you prepare the vegetables. Add the veggies as you chop them, adding them in the order listed. Add the seasonings and simmer until the potatoes are tender, about 45 minutes.

Makes 4-6 servings

Nutritional Analysis: One serving equals: 281.2 calories, 2.4g fat, 677mg sodium, 58.2g carbohydrate, 11g fiber, and 11g protein

Amazing Kale and Pinto Bean Soup

For most of my life I've thought that Kale existed solely to fill in the gaps between items at the salad bar. Come to find out that Kale is one amazing Superfood — it's packed with vitamins, minerals and cancer-fighting enzymes. It contains loads of vitamin A, vitamin C, B6, manganese, calcium, copper and potassium.

In addition to drinking Kale every morning in our green smoothie, I'm finding ways to include Kale at other meals. This soup is really easy to make. For a heartier soup, serve it over a scoop of cooked quinoa or brown rice.

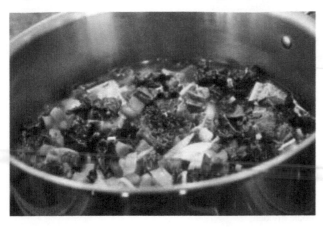

Here's what you need:

- 1 cup dried pinto beans
- 1 large yellow onion
- 1 Tablespoon olive oil
- 4 cloves garlic, minced
- 4 cups filtered water
- 2 vegan bouillon cubes (I use Rapunzel brand with sea salt and herbs)
- dash of freshly ground sea salt
- dash of freshly ground pepper
- 2 bay leaves
- 2 teaspoons dried rosemary, crushed between your fingers
- 5 large carrots, diced
- 2 bunches kale, chopped

1. Bring a large pot of water to a boil, add the beans and cook for 60-90 minutes. Drain and set aside.
2. In your soup pot heat the olive oil over medium heat. Add onion and garlic and cook for 5 minutes.
3. Add the cooked beans, water, bouillon, salt, pepper, bay leaves, rosemary, and carrots. Simmer for 15-20 minutes. Add the kale and cook another 15 minutes or until kale is tender. Add more water if needed.
4. Remove the bay leaves, add more salt and pepper if needed.

Makes 4 servings

Nutritional Analysis: One serving equals: 181 calories, 5g fat, 640.7mg sodium, 41.2g carbohydrate, 18.3g fiber, and 11g protein

Saffron Moroccan Stew

This is the perfect meal for a cold winter day, and as an added bonus the house smells amazing while this stew is cooking. Saffron, as you may know, is the world's most expensive spice by weight. Doesn't that make your stew feel extra special? Enjoy this exotic treat over quinoa.

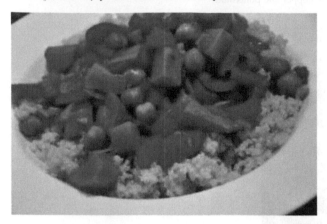

Here's what you need:

- 1 ½ cups plus 3 tablespoons water or vegetable stock, divided
- 1 large size yellow onion, finely chopped
- 2 large size red bell peppers, seeded and chopped
- 2 or 3 garlic cloves, minced
- 1 teaspoon Sucanat
- 1 teaspoon ground coriander
- ½ teaspoon ground cinnamon
- ½ teaspoon ground cumin
- 1 teaspoon grated or minced fresh ginger
- ½ teaspoon saffron threads (oooo and ahhhh over them before you throw them in the pot!)
- 2 medium size sweet potatoes or garnet or jewel yams, peeled and cut into ½ inch cubes
- 1 can (15oz) diced tomatoes, undrained
- 1 can (15oz) chickpeas drained and rinsed
- Salt and pepper to taste

1. Heat 3 tablespoons water in a soup pot over medium heat. Add onion, peppers and garlic, and cook for 5 minutes. If the water begins to evaporate, add a little more.
2. Stir in the Sucanat, coriander, cinnamon, cumin, ginger and saffron and cook for 1 minute, stirring constantly. Add sweet potatoes, and stir to coat. Stir in tomatoes, remaining 1 ½ cups water and chickpeas. Bring to a boil, then reduce heat to low.
3. Simmer until sweet potatoes are tender, about 30 minutes. Season with salt and pepper, then serve over quinoa

Makes 4 servings

Nutritional Analysis (without quinoa): One serving equals: 256.7 calories, 2.1g fat, 560.7mg sodium, 51g carbohydrate, 9.9g fiber, and 10.7g protein

Avocado Soup with Mango Salsa

Sometimes soup should be cold and refreshing, rather than hot and comforting. Avocado makes this soup amazingly creamy, and the salsa adds a nice kick of flavor.

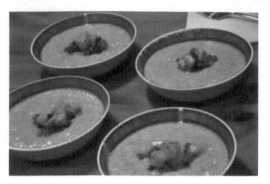

Here's what you need:

- 2 large cucumbers, chopped
- 2 large avocado, pitted and peeled
- 3 1/2 cups filtered water
- 2 green onions, chopped
- 1 celery stalk, chopped
- 1 lemon, squeezed
- 1 teaspoon ground cumin
- 1/4 teaspoon ground coriander
- 1 Tablespoon orange zest
- 1 bunch cilantro leaves
- 1 Tablespoon freshly ground sea salt

For the Salsa:

- 1 mango, chopped
- 1 yellow bell pepper, chopped
- 2 green heirloom tomatoes, chopped
- 2 mandarin oranges, chopped
- handful of cilantro, chopped
- handful of cherry tomatoes, chopped
- Freshly ground sea salt to taste

1. For the soup: Combine all of the ingredients in a high speed blender, mix until smooth
2. For the salsa: Combine all of the ingredients in a bowl, mix until fully combined.
3. Serve each bowl of soup with a large scoop of salsa.

Makes 4 servings

Nutritional Analysis: One serving equals: 272 calories, 15g fat, 1221mg sodium, 35.2g carbohydrate, 11.5g fiber, and 5g protein

White Bean Ratatouille

Ratatouille is a dish of cooked vegetables that originated in southern France, and this version contains loads of white beans which add protein and heartiness. Serve it hot or cold.

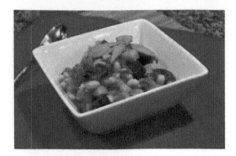

Here's what you need:

- 1 large-size globe eggplant, cut in ½ inch cubes
- 1 tablespoon water, for sautéing
- 2 medium-size red onions, sliced
- 3 medium-size zucchini, cut in ½ inch cubes
- 2 red bell peppers, cut into ½ inch squares
- 4 garlic cloves, minced
- ¼ cup dry white wine
- 1 cup vegetable stock
- 4 tomatoes, seeded and roughly chopped (or 2 cans – 15 oz each – fire roasted diced tomatoes)
- 1 tablespoon chopped fresh parsley
- ½ teaspoon dried thyme
- ½ teaspoon dried oregano
- 2 bay leaves
- 2 (15oz) cans white beans, drained and rinsed
- Salt and fresh group pepper, to taste
- ½ cup finely chopped fresh basil

1. Steam eggplant cubes for 10 minutes. Heat the water in a large-size sauté pan, add onions and cook, for 5 minutes.
2. Add zucchini and bell peppers and cook, stirring often, for another 5 minutes. Add steamed eggplant and cook another 5 minutes, then add garlic.
3. Add wine and stock. Bring to a boil over high heat, then reduce heat to medium-high and stir in tomatoes, parsley, thyme, oregano, and bay leaves. Reduce heat, cover, and simmer gently for 15 minutes, stirring occasionally.
4. Add beans to skillet, stirring well to combine. Cook, uncovered, until vegetables are tender but not mushy and liquids have thickened, stirring occasionally for another 5 minutes. Season with salt to taste.
5. Remove skillet from heat, remove the bay leaves, and stir in chopped basil.
6. Serve hot or cold.

Makes 4-6 servings

Nutritional Analysis: One serving equals: 351.2 calories, 3.5g fat, 1042mg sodium, 63.3g carbohydrate, 22.3g fiber, and 19.7g protein

Pumpkin and Quinoa with White Beans

This is another perfect dish for the holiday season. Quinoa is packed with protein and pumpkin is rich in antioxidants, vitamins and minerals.

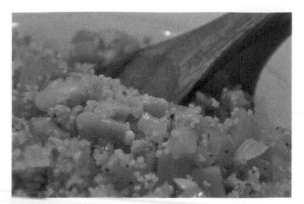

Here's what you need:

- 1 yellow onion, diced
- 6 celery stalks, diced
- 4 cups diced pumpkin
- 1 can white kidney beans, drained and rinsed
- 1 Tablespoon olive oil
- 1 Tablespoon fresh ginger, pressed
- 2 Tablespoon maple syrup
- dash of freshly ground sea salt
- zest and juice from 1 lemon
- 1/2 teaspoon ground cinnamon
- 1/4 teaspoon ground cardamom
- pinch of cloves
- pinch of nutmeg
- 2 cups filtered water
- 1 cup quinoa

1. Preheat oven to 400 degrees.
2. Place the onions, celery, beans and pumpkin in a large bowl. Mix in the oil, ginger and syrup, then sprinkle the salt and lemon zest. Add all the spices Mix until well combined and then place on a shallow baking dish. Cover the dish and bake for 40 minutes. After 40 minutes remove cover and cook for another 15 minutes.
3. While the vegetables are in the oven, put the quinoa and water in a saucepan, cover and bring to a boil over medium heat. Cook for about 25 minutes over low heat, until the water is absorbed.
4. Combine the vegetables and cooked quinoa together with the lemon juice. Serve warm or chilled.

Makes 4 servings

Nutritional Analysis: One serving equals: 385.7 calories, 7.2g fat, 531.7mg sodium, 68.4g carbohydrate, 11.5g fiber, and 16g protein

Real Healthy Stuffed Eggplant

Roasting veggies is a great way to keep it low fat and low calorie while adding delicious flavor and texture.

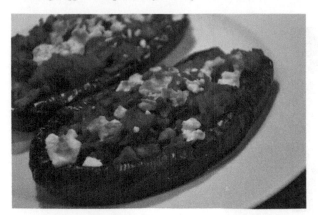

Here's what you need:

- 3 medium eggplants
- 1 teaspoon olive oil
- 2 medium onions, diced
- 2 cups cherry tomatoes, halved
- ¼ cup walnuts, chopped
- 2 teaspoons ground cinnamon
- 2 teaspoons dried oregano
- 1/4 cup reduced-fat feta cheese

1. Cut the eggplants in half, lengthwise, and scoop out the flesh, leaving ½ inch on the shell. Chop the scooped-out flesh into ½ inch cubes and set in a colander. Sprinkle the eggplant cubes and the inside of the eggplant shells with salt. Let stand for 30 minutes, then rinse and pat dry.
2. Bring a large pot of salted water to boil. Drop the eggplant shells in the water and simmer for 7 minutes. Shells should be barely tender when poked with a fork. Drain and pat dry.
3. Heat the olive oil in a large skillet over medium heat. Sauté the onions for 5 minutes. Add the chopped eggplant, tomatoes, walnuts, cinnamon, oregano and ¼ cup filtered water. Cook for 8 minutes, until softened and browned.
4. Preheat oven to broil. Place eggplant shells on a greased baking sheet. Broil for 5 minutes. Reduce oven heat to 375 degrees F.
5. Fill each eggplant shell with the veggies, sprinkle with the feta. Bake for 35 minutes, or until browned on top.

Makes 6 servings

Nutritional Analysis: One serving equals: 153 calories, 4.7g fat, 86mg sodium, 25g carbohydrate, 11g fiber, and 6g protein.

Real Healthy Eggplant Parmesan

Eggplant Parmesan is classic comfort food…but did you know that a dinner portion ordered at your favorite restaurant contains more than 1,000 calories and 60 grams of fat?!?! There's nothing comforting about that.

This recipe for Real Healthy Eggplant Parmesan has been significantly lightened. I've eliminated the fryer and the white flour, resulting in a tender and tasty dish that won't land on your hips.

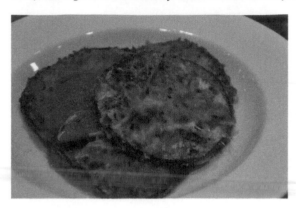

Here's what you need for 10 servings:

- 2 medium, organic eggplants
- 1 1/2 cup blanched almond flour
- 1 teaspoon salt
- 1 teaspoon dried basil
- 1 Tablespoon flax meal
- 2 omega-3, free range eggs
- 2 Tablespoons filtered water
- 1 Tablespoon olive oil
- 3 cups organic spaghetti sauce
- 1 cup shredded mozzarella cheese
- 1/4 cup grated Parmesan cheese

1. Preheat the oven to 350 degrees F.
2. Slice the eggplant into slices no larger than 1/4 inch.
3. In a medium bowl combine the almond flour, salt, basil and flax. In another medium bowl whisk the eggs and water. Dip each slice of eggplant in the egg mixture and then coat each side with the almond flour mixture.
4. Place a large skillet over medium heat. Coat with the olive oil. Saute the eggplant slices until tender and golden, about 5 minutes per side. Transfer to a paper towel-lined plate.
5. Spread 1 cup of the spaghetti sauce into a 13×9 baking pan. Place a layer of eggplant over the sauce, then sprinkle 1/2 cup of the mozzarella evenly over it. Cover with another cup of spaghetti sauce and another layer of eggplant. Top with the remaining sauce, mozzarella and Parmesan cheese.
6. Cover with foil, bake for 20 minutes. Remove foil and turn the oven to broil for 3-5 minutes, until the top is browned.

Makes 10 Servings

Nutritional Analysis: One serving equals: 205 calories, 13g fat, 518mg sodium, 15g carbohydrate, 6g fiber, and 9g protein.

Real Healthy Zucchini Cakes

This recipe is very light, with no potato or gluten weighing it down. Top it with a dollop of plain Greek yogurt and a sprinkle of sweet paprika.

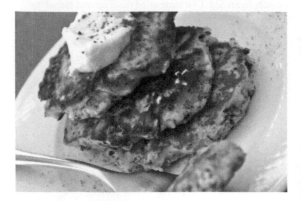

Here's what you need:

- 1 tsp olive oil
- 1 small yellow onion, grated
- 1 garlic clove
- 2 cups grated Zucchini
- 1/2 tsp salt
- 2 eggs
- 1/4 cup coconut flour
- 2 Tablespoons flax meal
- 1/2 tsp baking powder
- Non-Fat Plain Greek Yogurt
- Sweet Paprika

1. Heat half of the olive oil in a large skillet. Saute the onion and garlic for 2 minutes, then set aside.
2. Place grated zucchini in a colander, sprinkle with the salt and allow to sit in the sink for 10 minutes.
3. Use a clean paper towel to squeeze excess water from the zucchini.
4. In a medium sized bowl whisk the eggs. Add the coconut flour, flax and baking powder. Add the onions and zucchini.
5. Place the remaining olive oil in a large skillet over medium heat. Drop the dough in heaping Tablespoons, press down with a fork. Cook each side for 3 minutes or until golden.
6. Serve with a dollop of yogurt and a sprinkle of sweet paprika.

Makes 8 Servings

Nutritional Analysis: One serving equals: 51 calories, 2.7g fat, 188mg sodium, 4g carbohydrate, 2g fiber, and 3g protein.

Best Spaghetti Squash Casserole

This casserole is a perfect replacement for heavy pasta dishes that leave you feeling sluggish. Spaghetti squash contains omega-3 essential fatty acids, good for preventing heart disease, cancer and inflammation caused by arthritis, and omega-6 fatty acids which promotes brain function. Imagine that — a 'pasta' dish that is packed with many vitamins and minerals, which are required for proper functioning of the body. Almost too good to be true.

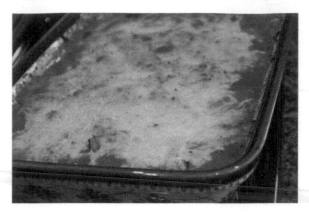

Here's what you need:

- 1 spaghetti squash
- 1 tablespoon olive oil
- 3 cloves garlic
- 1 sweet onion, chopped
- 2 zucchini, chopped
- 2 medium tomatoes, chopped
- 1/3 cup basil leaves, chopped
- 2 teaspoons dried oregano
- 1 jar organic spaghetti sauce
- Shredded soy cheese

1. Preheat oven to 400 degrees F.
2. Cut spaghetti squash in half. Scoop out the seeds. Splash inside of squash with water, then microwave each half individually for 5 minutes. Careful when removing from microwave — it will be hot. Set aside to cool.
3. Heat olive oil in a large skillet over medium heat. Add garlic. After a few minutes add onion. After a few minutes add zucchini. Finally add tomatoes, basil and oregano and cook for another 5 minutes, until everything is tender.
4. Scoop out the spaghetti squash and place in a large mixing bowl. Add the veggies from skillet. Pour the entire jar of spaghetti squash into the bowl and mix well.
5. Place the squash mixture in a large casserole dish, top with cheese and bake for 20-25 minutes, until the cheese is golden.

Makes 8 servings

Nutritional Analysis: One serving equals: 161.5 calories, 6.2 fat, 523mg sodium, 20.8g carbohydrate, 5.3g fiber, and 8.4g protein.

Real Healthy Sweet Potato Casserole

Why do sweet potatoes always seem to get saddled with marshmallows during the holidays? This recipe is the perfect alternative to extra-sugary sweet potato casseroles. I cook this in a large skillet, which is nice when the ovens are taken up with so many other holiday dishes.

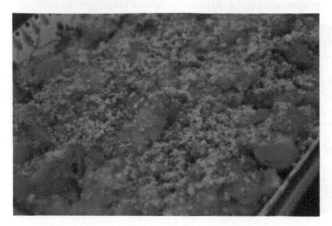

Here's what you need:

- 1 Tablespoon coconut oil
- 6 sweet potatoes, peeled and cut into small cubes
- 1 cup vegetable broth
- 1/4 cup pure maple syrup
- dash of salt and pepper
- Juice from 1 lime
- 1 cup ground walnuts

1. Heat the coconut oil in a large skillet.
2. Add the sweet potato cubes and cook, stirring occasionally, until lightly browned — about 10 minutes.
3. Add the broth, maple syrup salt, pepper and lime juice. Bring to a boil.
4. Reduce to a simmer and cover for 10 minutes. Remove cover and continue to cook, stirring occasionally until all liquid is absorbed.
5. Transfer to a casserole dish. Evenly sprinkle the ground walnuts on top.
6. *Optional* If you want the walnuts to be toasty then place in the oven on broil for a few minutes.

Makes 8 servings

Nutritional Analysis: One serving equals: 238.6 calories, 11.5 fat, 131.2mg sodium, 33.7g carbohydrate, 4.1g fiber, and 3.7g protein.

Tempeh and Veggie Stir Fry

What a great way to cook veggies and tempeh! If you're not into tempeh feel free to leave it out or to replace it with firm or baked tofu or seitan. The veggies below are just a guide — really any of the veggies that you have on hand would work beautifully!

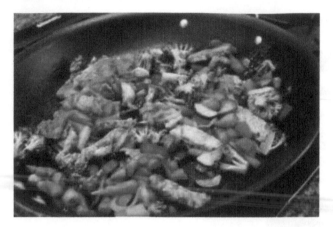

Here's what you need:

- 1 Tablespoon sesame oil
- 1 onion, cut in half and then sliced
- 1 (8 oz) package organic 5-grain tempeh, thinly sliced and halved
- 2 small zucchini, cut in half lengthwise and thinly sliced
- 1 1/2 cup carrots, sliced
- 1 Tablespoon Nama shoyu (or Tamari or soy sauce)
- 2 cups broccoli florets
- 2 teaspoons toasted sesame oil

1. Heat the sesame oil in a large skillet. Throw in the onions, cook for a few minutes. Add the tempeh, cook for a few more minutes. Add the zucchini and cook for another few minutes.
2. Place the carrots on top of the veggies in the skillet, add 1/4 cup of water, cover and simmer for 7 minutes. Add the shoyu and broccoli to the pan, cover and simmer for another 5 minutes.
3. Remove from heat, drizzle with toasted sesame oil and mix to coat.

Makes 4 servings

Nutritional Analysis: One serving equals: 238.2 calories, 11.6 fat, 300mg sodium, 23g carbohydrate, 9.3g fiber, and 13.6g protein.

Teriyaki Tofu

This is a wonderful recipe for tofu newbies. It is simple, quick and always tastes delicious. There is virtually no way to mess up this recipe (unless you accidentally leave it in the oven for an extra hour and burn it—but you won't do that).

Serve your teriyaki tofu up on brown or wild rice, with quinoa or even on a bed of greens. Leftovers are perfect for adding to sandwiches, wraps or salads.

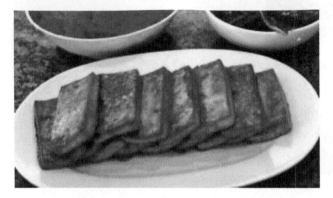

Here's what you need:

- 12 oz package of organic firm tofu *If you're feeding more than 2 people I'd do at least 2 12oz packages

- 1 Tablespoon peanut oil
- California Teriyaki Marinade, Consorzio by Annie's Naturals

1. Preheat oven to 350.
2. Drain and press your tofu, then slice it.
3. Coat a 9"x13" glass pan or cookie sheet with the peanut oil, place the tofu slices on the bottom of the pan, turning them once to coat both sides.
4. Bake for 15 minutes. Remove from oven, turn each slice over, then return to oven for an additional 15 minutes.
5. Remove from oven, pour the teriyaki marinade over the tofu slices, turning them to coat both sides. Return to oven for a final 15 minutes.
6. Serve and enjoy!

Makes 4 servings

Nutritional Analysis: One serving equals: 211.2 calories, 11g fat, 393mg sodium, 13.7g carbohydrate, 1.3g fiber, and 15g protein.

Moroccan Salmon with Braised Kale

Here's a new take on salmon that is tasty and super quick to make. The savory yogurt and tender kale go perfectly together.

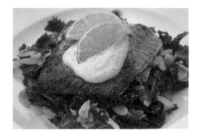

For the Salmon:

- 1/2 cup Greek yogurt, fat free
- 1 lime, juiced
- 1 Tablespoon olive oil
- 3 garlic cloves, minced (or 3 frozen minced garlic cubes from Trader Joe's)
- 1 1/2 teaspoons ground coriander
- 1 1/2 teaspoons ground cumin
- 4 (6oz) wild caught salmon fillets

For the Kale:

- 1/2 cup sliced almonds
- 1 Tablespoon organic butter
- 1 yellow onion, chopped
- 1 (10oz) bag kale, chopped (or 1 large bunch kale chopped)
- 1/2 cup hot water
- 1 vegetable bouillon
- dash of freshly ground pepper
- dash of freshly ground salt

1. Preheat oven to 375 degrees F. Coat a baking pan with nonstick spray and set aside.
2. In a small bowl combine the yogurt, lime juice, garlic, spices, salt and pepper. Put half of the yogurt mixture aside in the fridge. Coat the salmon with the other half of the yogurt mixture and marinate in the fridge for 30 minutes.
3. While the salmon marinates, place a large skillet over medium heat. Add the almonds and toast for 5 minutes, until golden. Add the butter and allow to brown. Add the garlic and onions and cook for another 5 minutes.
4. Dissolve the bouillon in the water and then add to the skillet. Cook for another 10 minutes until tender and the liquid has evaporated.
5. Place the salmon on prepared pan and bake for 20 minutes. Turn on the high broil for an additional 5 minutes until the top of the salmon has browned.
6. Serve the salmon on a bed of kale with a dollop of the reserved yogurt.

Makes 8 servings

Nutritional Analysis: One serving equals: 416.7 calories, 23.1g fat, 253mg sodium, 9.3g carbohydrate, 2.8g fiber, and 45.2g protein.

15 Minute Tropical Fish Tacos

I love love love fast recipes for healthy fast dinners. Try the marinated frozen cod from Trader Joe's — it was a huge hit with the whole family. Simply put the frozen fillets in the fridge the night before or in the morning, and the rest of the meal comes together in 15 minutes flat.

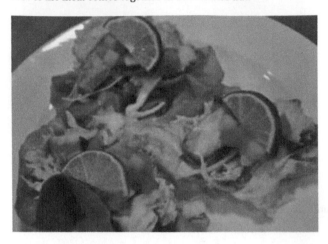

Here's what you need:

- Wild Marinated Soy Ginger Cod Fillets, Trader Joe's
- 1 lime
- 1 head living lettuce
- Guacamole, buy pre-made
- 1 cup shredded cabbage, buy pre-shredded
- Papaya mango salsa, Trader Joe's has a good one

1. Defrost frozen cod by placing in the fridge overnight.
2. Preheat oven to 375 degrees F. Grease a pan with olive oil.
3. Place defrosted cod in prepared pan, cut lime in half and squeeze juice over cod. Bake for 15 minutes.
4. While cod is baking, separate leaves from lettuce, being careful to keep them intact. Assemble individual tacos by putting a tablespoon of guacamole on a lettuce leaf, topped with a sprinkle of cabbage.
5. Once fish is done, change oven to broil for a few minutes, watching closely until top is browned. Remove from oven and cut into 1 inch pieces.
6. Top each prepared taco with a piece of fish, a spoonful of salsa, and a slice of the remaining lime half.

Makes 4 servings

Nutritional Analysis: One serving equals: 246.2 calories, 12.6g fat, 602mg sodium, 16g carbohydrate, 3.9g fiber, and 19g protein.

Real Healthy Fish Sticks

Fish sticks are a childhood food staple, but who really wants to feed their kids a dinner that's been battered and fried? This recipe gives you all the crispiness that kids love without the grease. Serve with a side of veggies and some tartar sauce.

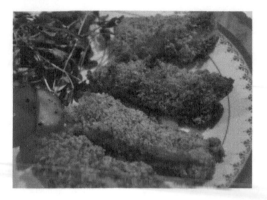

Here's what you need:

- Olive oil
- 18 oz white fish fillet, cut into strips
- 1/3 cup coconut flour
- 1 teaspoon garlic salt
- dash of pepper
- 1/2 cup almond meal
- 1/2 cup ground walnuts
- 2 organic, free range eggs

1. Preheat oven to 450 degrees F. Prepare a baking sheet by drizzling with olive oil and coating evenly. Set aside.
2. In a small bowl combine the coconut flour, garlic salt and pepper. In another small bowl combine the almond meal and ground walnuts. In a third small bowl whisk the eggs until frothy.
3. Take each strip of fish and dredge it in the flour mixture, then dip in the egg, and then coat with the ground nuts. Place on prepared pan.
4. Bake for 20 minutes or until golden and crispy.

Makes 4 servings

Nutritional Analysis: One serving equals: 278.7 calories, 14.3g fat, 443mg sodium, 6g carbohydrate, 3.3g fiber, and 32.1g protein.

Mango Chutney Smothered Mahi Mahi on Sauteed Cabbage

If I were to ever open a restaurant, this recipe would be the star of the menu. Delicately seasoned Mahi Mahi is complemented perfectly by the richly flavorful chutney and mild sauteed cabbage. The entire process take only an hour, and it is SO worth the effort!

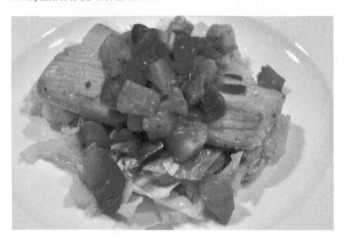

Here's what you need:

For the Mahi Mahi:

- juice from 1 lemon
- 1/4 cup olive oil
- 1 teaspoon salt
- 1 teaspoon pepper
- dash of red pepper flakes
- 4 cloves garlic (or 4 frozen minced garlic cubes from Trader Joe's)
- 4 Wild caught Mahi Mahi fillets (I buy mine from freezer section in Trader Joe's)

1. Place all ingredients, except the fish, in a high speed blender. Blend until fully combined.
2. Combine the marinade with fillets in a large ziplock bag. Place in the fridge for 60 minutes.
3. Preheat oven to 450 degrees F, if fish is frozen; or 375 degrees F, if fish is thawed.
4. Grease a pan and place fish fillets on it. For frozen fish, bake for 12-20 minutes, until fish is opaque and flakes easily. For thawed fish, bake for 6 minutes, then flip and bake for additional 6 minutes.

For the Chutney:

- 1 Tablespoon coconut oil
- 2 cloves garlic, minced (or 2 frozen minced garlic cubes from Trader Joe's)
- 1 inch ginger root, minced
- 1 small red onion, chopped
- 1 small red bell pepper, chopped
- 1 small green bell pepper, chopped
- 3 ripe mangoes, chopped (don't worry if your mangoes aren't the sweetest — once cooked it tastes much sweeter)
- juice from 2 limes
- 1 Tablespoon curry powder

- 1 teaspoon ground cinnamon
- dash of nutmeg
- dash of red pepper flakes

1. In a large skillet, heat coconut oil over medium heat. Add garlic and ginger root and saute for a minute.
2. Add the onion and bell peppers and saute for a few minutes.
3. Add the mango and spices. Continue to saute for another 5 minutes, until everything has softened.
4. Turn the heat down to low, cover and simmer for another 10 minutes.

For the Sauteed Cabbage:

- 1 small green cabbage
- 1 Tablespoon coconut oil
- dash of salt
- dash of pepper

1. Wash cabbage and discard the first few leaves. Slice it thinly.
2. Place a large skillet on medium heat. Add the coconut oil, and once that melts, add the cabbage.
3. Sprinkle with salt and pepper, and cook for 5 minutes, stirring frequently.

To Serve:

1. Arrange each plate with a bed of cabbage, then top with a fillet smothered in chutney.

Makes 4-6 servings

Nutritional Analysis: One serving equals: 400 calories, 14.8g fat, 217mg sodium, 47g carbohydrate, 10.5g fiber, and 25.8g protein.

Agave Teriyaki Salmon

During a trip to Kauai we picked up an amazing recipe for teriyaki salmon from Roy's restaurant. It's been more than 10 years since that trip but the recipe just never gets old. I've modified the recipe to use agave nectar instead of refined white sugar, and honestly think it tastes better than the original.

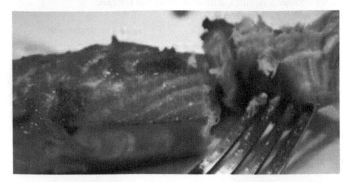

Here's what you need:

- Wild caught salmon fillet
- 1 cup soy sauce
- 1/4 cup agave nectar
- 3 Tablespoons minced garlic
- 3 Tablespoons minced ginger root

1. Combine all ingredients in a large ziplock bag. Allow to marinate in fridge for 40-60 minutes.
2. Preheat oven to 350 degrees F. Remove salmon fillet from marinade and place in a large glass pan. Strain the minced garlic and ginger pieces from marinade and arrange on the fillet. Bake for 20 minutes. Turn on broiler for additional 5 minutes.

Makes 2 servings

Nutritional Analysis: One serving equals: 350 calories, 6.2g fat, 811mg sodium, 38g carbohydrate, 1.3g fiber, and 39g protein.

Real Healthy Fried Chicken

Excuse me, but who said that eating healthy meant only eating green things? I, for one, oppose that idea. Sure, salads are great…but not for every meal. I believe in eating everything that we want – and with just a few modifications we can make it healthier. For example…fried chicken. Who doesn't enjoy the crispy, crunchy, satisfying morsels? This recipe takes fried chicken to a happy, healthy place.

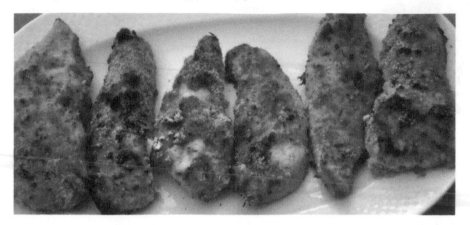

Here's what you need:

- 2 eggs
- 2 Tablespoons fruit-only apricot preserves
- 2 Tablespoons Dijon mustard
- 1/2 teaspoon garlic powder
- 1/2 teaspoon red pepper flakes
- 1/2 cup almond flour
- 1/2 cup almond meal
- 1/2 cup coconut flour
- 1/2 teaspoon black pepper
- 1/2 teaspoon dried thyme
- 1/2 teaspoon sweet paprika
- 1/2 teaspoon salt
- 2 lbs boneless, skinless organic chicken tenders

1. Preheat oven to 350 degrees F. Lightly grease a 13″x9″ baking pan with coconut oil.
2. In a medium bowl whisk the eggs, apricot preserves, mustard, garlic powder, and red pepper flakes.
3. In another medium bowl combine the almond flour, almond meal, coconut flour, pepper, thyme, paprika and salt.
4. Dip each chicken tender in the egg mixture, then dredge through the flour mixture. Place in the prepared pan.
5. Bake for 35 minutes. Change oven to high broil for 2 minutes, flip each chicken tender and broil the other side for 2 minutes.
6. Serve with a side of sugar-free BBQ sauce or organic honey mustard.

Makes 6 Servings

Nutritional Analysis: One serving equals: 256 calories, 6g fat, 376mg sodium, 5g carbohydrate, 2g fiber, and 39g protein.

Southwest Stuffed Chicken

This dish is savory with the rich flavors of the Southwest. It's the perfect dish to make if you're in a boring grilled chicken breast rut.

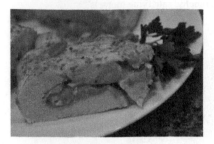

Here's what you need:

- 4 oz light cream cheese, room temperature
- 1 (15oz) can diced tomatoes, drained
- 1/2 cup frozen corn kernels
- 1 (4oz) can Hatch green chiles, roasted and chopped
- Salt and pepper
- 4 organic, boneless, skinless chicken breasts
- Olive oil
- Tajin seasoning (blend of dehydrated lime, ground chile peppers and salt)

1. Preheat oven to 350 degrees F.
2. In a medium bowl with an electric mixer on low speed, combine the cream cheese, drained tomatoes, corn and chiles.
3. Slice through the thick part of each chicken breast so that it opens like a book. Double wrap the chicken with plastic wrap and out it with a meat mallet (really good activity for stress relief!) until it's 1/2 to 1/4 inches thick.
4. Season one side of each chicken breast with salt and pepper, then flip it over and spread with 1/4 of the cream cheese filling. Roll each chicken breast up and place it seam side down in a baking dish. Rub a little olive oil over the top of the chicken then season with Tajin and salt and pepper.
5. Cover and bake for 35 minutes. Remove the cover and bake for another 15 minutes.
6. Thinly slice and then serve.

Makes 4 Servings

Nutritional Analysis: One serving equals: 242 calories, 7g fat, 549mg sodium, 10g carbohydrate, 3g fiber, and 34g protein.

Turkey-Stuffed Bell Peppers

Eating healthy does not have to be boring! These turkey-stuffed bell peppers are the perfect meal for those days when you're just sick and tired of eating healthy. Shhhh, your taste buds will never know that this dish is low-carb and protein-filled. Serve over a bed of greens for a complete meal.

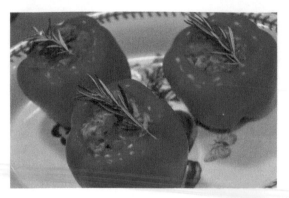

Here's what you need for 5 bell peppers:

- 5 organic bell peppers
- 1 Tablespoon olive oil
- 2 cloves garlic (or 2 frozen minced garlic cubes from Trader Joe's)
- 2 Tablespoons fresh basil, minced (or 2 frozen minced basil cubes from Trader Joe's)
- 1 yellow onion, minced
- 1 Tablespoon fresh rosemary, minced
- 1 teaspoon dried parsley
- dash of salt and pepper
- 20 oz organic ground turkey
- 1 organic tomato, chopped
- 3/4 cup spaghetti sauce
- 1/2 cup shredded mozzarella cheese

1. Bring a large pot of water to boil, add a pinch of salt. Cut the tops off the bell peppers and remove the seeds. Place in the boiling water, using a spoon to keep them submerged for 3 minutes or until the skin is slightly softened. Drain and set aside.
2. Preheat the oven to 350 degrees F. Prepare a baking pan with non-stick cooking spray and set aside.
3. In a large skillet heat the oil on medium. Add the garlic, basil, onion, rosemary, parsley, salt and pepper. Cook for about 5 minutes, until the onions begin to soften. Add the ground turkey and continue to heat until the meat is browned. Add the tomato and cook for another 2 minutes.
4. Remove from heat. Pour the spaghetti sauce into the turkey mixture and mix well. Add the cheese and mix until well combined.
5. Stuff each prepared bell pepper with the turkey mixture and place on prepared baking sheet. Cook for 15-20 minutes until the bell peppers are tender.

Makes 5 servings

Nutritional Analysis: One serving equals: 294 calories, 14g fat, 347mg sodium, 15.5g carbohydrate, 3.8g fiber, and 27.5g protein.

Real Healthy Pizza

Here is a healthy twist on pizza that allows you to enjoy your favorite flavors without going into carb-overload. This simple crust is made with eggs in a skillet.

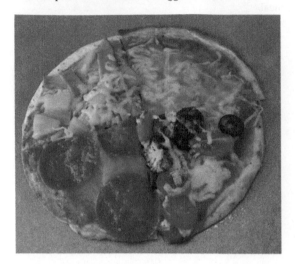

Here's what you need for 1 individual pizza:

- 3 eggs
- dash of salt and pepper
- non-stick cooking spray
- 2 Tablespoons pizza sauce
- 1/4 cup shredded mozzarella cheese
- Toppings of your choice: Canadian bacon, pineapple, pepperoni, olives, broccoli, tomatoes…

1. Preheat your oven to high broil and position a rack at the very top position. Spray a baking sheet with non-stick cooking spray and set aside.
2. Place two skillets on medium heat — the perfect size is about a 7 inch diameter– and spray both with non-stick spray.
3. Whisk the eggs, salt and pepper until well combined. Pour into one of the prepared skillets, place a lid on, and cook for about 3 minutes.
4. **Don't move the eggs around** When the eggs are set remove the lid and flip it into the other prepared skillet to cook the other side. This method works perfectly for creating an egg crust that is intact and strong. Cook for about a minute, then flip the egg crust onto the prepared baking sheet.
5. Spread the crust with sauce, sprinkle with cheese and add your toppings. Place in the oven under high broil for exactly 1 minute and 30 seconds.
6. Remove from oven and enjoy.

Makes 1-2 servings

Nutritional Analysis (without toppings): One serving equals: 319 calories, 20.7g fat, 500mg sodium, 5.8g carbohydrate, .5g fiber, and 26.9g protein.

Garden Medley with Apple Sausage

Spaghetti squash replaces noodles in this low carb casserole with lots of other veggies added for extra fiber, vitamins and flavor. Organic apple sausage is filled with protein, making this the perfect complete meal.

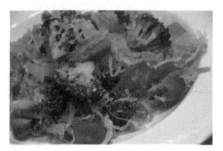

Here's what you need:

- 1 medium sized spaghetti squash
- 1 teaspoon olive oil
- 2 cloves garlic minced (or 2 frozen cubes from Trader Joes)
- 1 medium onion, chopped
- 1 cup shredded carrots
- 1 cup sliced mushrooms
- 1 bunch broccoli, chopped
- 12 oz organic sausage, sliced (try Niman Ranch Apple Gouda Sausage)
- dash of salt and pepper
- 1/4 cup kalamata olives, chopped
- 1 cup heirloom cherry tomatoes, halved
- 1/2 cup shredded organic cheese
- 1 cup Organic spaghetti sauce

1. Preheat oven to 325 degrees F.
2. Cut the squash in half. Scoop out the seeds. Fill a microwave safe dish with an inch of water, and place half of the squash in it, cut side down. Microwave for 10 minutes (OR place oven safe pan with an inch of water into the oven at 350 for 40 minutes). Carefully remove from microwave (will be hot). Repeat with the other half. Put aside to cool.
3. In a large skillet heat the olive oil on medium. Add garlic. Add the onions and cook for about 3 minutes. Add the shredded carrots and mushrooms. After a few minutes toss the broccoli pieces on top and cover for 5 minutes. Remove cover, stir and cook for another minute until the veggies are all tender.
4. In a medium skillet, heat the sliced sausage over medium heat. Once browned, remove from heat.
5. In a large bowl scrape out the insides of the spaghetti squash and discard the skin. Add the veggies and sausage. Add a dash of salt and pepper. Add olives and tomatoes.
6. Lightly grease a large casserole pan with olive oil. Evenly press the veggie and sausage mixture into the pan. Top with shredded cheese.
7. Bake for 25 minutes or until bubbly.
8. Serve with a spoonful of spaghetti sauce.

Makes 6 servings

Nutritional Analysis: One serving equals: 200 calories, 6.5g fat, 464mg sodium, 24g carbohydrate, 6.7g fiber, and 14g protein.

Easy Apple Pork Chops

I love easy, nutritious recipes like this that come together quickly.

Putting apples and onions with pork chops and then smothering it in cinnamon creates a surprisingly delicious, healthy meal.

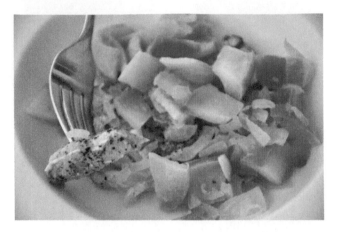

Here's what you need for 4 servings:

- 2 apples, chopped
- 1 medium yellow onion, chopped
- 2 Tablespoons coconut oil
- cinnamon
- sea salt
- 4 lean pork chops
- 1/4 cup white wine
- 1/4 cup sliced almonds

1. In a large skillet warm 1 Tablespoon of the coconut oil over medium heat. Add the apples and onions. Saute for 5 minutes until the apples are tender.
2. Remove the apples and onions from the pan.
3. Add the remaining Tablespoon of coconut oil to the pan and leave the heat on medium. Sprinkle cinnamon and salt on both sides of the pork chops then rub in.
4. Place the pork chops in the pan, sear on each side for 2 minutes.
5. Add the wine and bring to a boil. Add the apples and onions back to the pan, cover and cook for about 6 minutes.
6. Sprinkle with the almonds and serve the chops with a generous helping of the apples and onions.

4 Servings

Nutritional Analysis: One serving equals: 296 calories, 12g fat, 94mg sodium, 10g carbohydrate, 2g fiber, and 21g protein

Real Healthy Zucchini Brownies

Hmmmmm, what to do with all the zucchini from the garden? Make brownies?!? Yes! This recipe is so much fun, Zucchini adds moisture and is virtually undetectable.

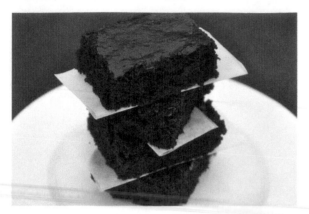

Here's what you need:

- 5 oz dark chocolate, 72% or higher cocoa content
- 1/4 cup coconut oil
- 2 omega-3, free range eggs
- 1/4 cup agave nectar
- 2 teaspoons vanilla extract
- 1/4 teaspoon almond extract
- 1 cup blanched almond flour
- 1/4 cup unsweetened cocoa powder
- 1 1/2 teaspoons baking soda
- 1/4 teaspoon salt
- 1 1/2 cups shredded zucchini

1. Preheat oven to 350 degrees F. Grease an 8×8 pan with coconut oil, then dust with blanched almond flour. Set aside.
2. In a double boiler, gently melt the chocolate. (If you don't have a double boiler then fill a skillet with a few inches of water and set a small pot in the water, place over very low heat.) Add the coconut oil and mix until fully combined. Remove from heat and set aside to cool.
3. In small bowl combine the eggs, agave nectar and vanilla and almond extracts. Add the cooled chocolate mixture.
4. In a medium bowl combine almond flour, cocoa powder, baking soda and salt. Pour in the wet ingredients and mix until fully combined.
5. Using a food processor, shred the zucchini. Then place on a cutting board and finely chop the shredded pieces. Having very tiny pieces of zucchini is the key to making this recipe work!
6. Fold the zucchini into the batter. Pour into prepared pan and bake for 25 minutes, or until fully set. Allow to cool in the pan for at least 30 minutes before cutting. *Tip: Use a serrated, plastic knife to cut your brownies — this makes it less likely to crumble.

Makes 16 servings

Nutritional Analysis: One serving equals: 116 calories, 8g fat, 102mg sodium, 7g carbohydrate, 2g fiber, and 3g protein.

Black Bean Brownies

To the naked eye these look like any other scrumptious chocolate brownie, but on the inside they are filled with protein and fiber rich black beans. And they taste amazing.

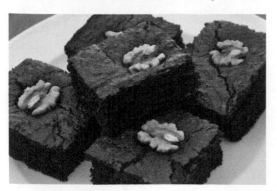

Here's what you need:

- 1 1/2 cup almond meal (ground almonds)
- 1 1/2 teaspoon baking soda
- 1 1/2 teaspoon baking powder
- 1/2 teaspoon sea salt
- 1 can beans (15oz), drained
- 1 cup melted dark chocolate (72% cocoa or higher)
- 1/3 cup melted coconut oil
- 1/2 cup melted raw honey
- 2 teaspoons vanilla extract
- 1/4 teaspoon almond extract
- 2 organic, omega-3 eggs
- 12 walnut halves

1. Preheat oven to 350 degrees F. Lightly grease a brownie pan with coconut oil. Set aside.
2. In a medium bowl combine the almond meal, baking soda, baking powder and salt.
3. In a high speed blender combine the drained beans, melted chocolate, coconut oil, honey, vanilla and almond extracts. Blend on low speed until smooth.
4. Pour the wet ingredients into the bowl of dry ingredients and mix. Add the eggs and mix until fully incorporated.
5. Pour into prepared pan. Place the walnut halves on top.
6. Bake for 25-30 minutes. Allow to cool fully before cutting into squares.

Makes 30 servings

Nutritional Analysis: One serving equals: 147.7 calories, 9.8g fat, 87mg sodium, 12.9g carbohydrate, 2.5g fiber, and 3.3g protein.

Skinny Lemon Bars

Biting into a Skinny Lemon Bar is like turning back the hands of time to revisit what it felt like to not care how productive a day would be, but to simply care about enjoying the moment. With no refined sugar or flour, you can enjoy the delicately sweet treat without worrying about adding an extra workout.

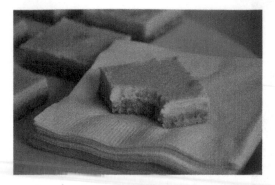

For the Crust:

- 3 cups blanched almond flour
- 1 teaspoon salt
- 1/4 cup coconut oil, melted over low heat
- 2 Tablespoons agave nectar
- 1 Tablespoon vanilla extract
- 1/2 teaspoon almond extract
- 1 teaspoon lemon rind

For the Lemon Layer:

- 1/2 cup coconut oil, melted over low heat
- 1/2 cup agave nectar
- 6 omega-3, free range eggs
- 2/3 cup fresh lemon juice
- 2 Tablespoons lemon rind
- 2 Tablespoons coconut flour

1. Preheat oven to 350 degrees F. Generously grease a 13"x9" baking pan with coconut oil and lightly dust with coconut flour. Set aside.
2. For the crust: In a medium bowl combine the almond flour and salt. In another bowl combine the coconut oil, agave nectar, extracts and lemon rind. Mix the dry and wet ingredients together until well combined. Press the dough into the bottom of prepared pan. Bake for 15 minutes, or until golden.
3. For the Lemon Layer: In a blender combine all of the lemon layer ingredients on high until smooth. Pour over the baked crust. Bake for another 15-20 minutes until golden. Allow to cool for 30 minutes then refrigerate for 2 hours until set. Cut into bars and serve.

Makes 30 servings

Nutritional Analysis: One serving equals: 151.2 calories, 12.3g fat, 60mg sodium, 8.7g carbohydrate, 1.5g fiber, and 3.7g protein.

Real Healthy No-Bake Cookies

These easy no-bake cookies are perfect for sitting around enjoying tea and cookies with friends.

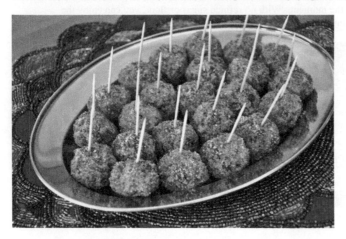

Here's what you need for 35 cookie balls:

- 1.5 cup almond flour, plus 1/4 cup for topping
- 1 cup mini chocolate chips
- 1/2 cup coconut crystals, plus 1/2 cup for topping
- 1/2 cup almond butter
- 1/4 cup coconut oil
- 1 cup unsweetened shredded coconut
- 2 tsp cinnamon

1. Line a baking sheet with wax paper. Set aside.
2. In a large bowl, combine the almond flour, chocolate chips, coconut crystals, almond butter, coconut oil, shredded coconut and cinnamon.
3. In a small bowl combine the almond flour and coconut crystals for the topping.
4. Form round balls out of 1 Tablespoon scoops of dough, roll in the topping, then place on prepared baking sheet.
5. Chill the cookie balls in the fridge for 30 minutes.

Makes 35 Servings

Nutritional Analysis: One serving equals: 145 calories, 11g fat, 10mg sodium, 8g carbohydrate, 2g fiber, and 4g protein.

Caveman Chocolate Chunk Cookies

These cookies are made with almond flour and crammed with macadamia nuts, making them high in fat. If you're still a fat-phobic (I certainly was in the 90's!) it's time to put down your fears and embrace healthy fats. Fat keeps you full for a long, long time. One of these little cookies will energize your entire afternoon.

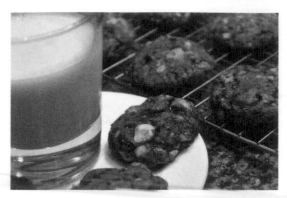

Here's what you need:

- 4 cups almond meal (1 full bag from Trader Joe's)
- 1 teaspoons baking soda
- 1/2 teaspoon salt
- 1/4 cup coconut oil
- 1/4 cup raw honey
- 2 omega-3 eggs
- 1 teaspoon vanilla extract
- 1 teaspoon almond extract
- 10 oz (2 cups) roasted, unsalted macadamia nuts, chopped or pulsed in food processor
- 2 (5oz) bars 72% cocoa baking chocolate, chopped or pulsed in food processor

1. Preheat oven to 350 degrees F. Line baking sheets with wax paper.
2. In a large bowl combine the almond meal, baking soda and salt. Mix well.
   Over low heat, in small saucepan, gently melt coconut oil and honey. Add to bowl. Add eggs and mix well. Add vanilla and almond extracts. Add macadamia nuts and chocolate. Mix until fully incorporated.
3. Shape dough into golf ball-sized balls, then flatten onto pan. Bake for 12-15 minutes until golden.
   Allow to cool before removing from pan.

Makes 30 cookies

Nutritional Analysis: One cookie equals: 224 calories, 19.2g fat, 108mg sodium, 9.8g carbohydrate, 3.2g fiber, and 4.7g protein.

Andrew's Flourless Walnut Cookies

If you're looking for a delicious treat that is also nutritious and provides energy for your mind and body, these Flourless Walnut Cookies will do the trick. These cookies are really tasty, and best of all it only takes 25 minutes from start to finish.

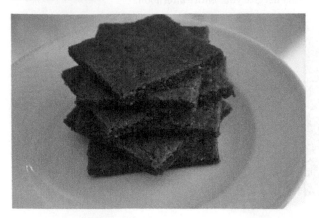

Here's what you need:

- 2 cups walnuts
- 1 teaspoon baking soda
- 3 teaspoons cinnamon
- 1/2 teaspoon nutmeg
- 1/2 teaspoon sea salt
- 2 tablespoons melted Earthbalance butter
- 1 tablespoon raw honey, melted
- 1 tablespoon water

1. Preheat oven to 375 degrees F. Line a cookie sheet with wax paper.
2. Place the walnuts, baking soda, salt, cinnamon, and nutmeg in a food processor. Pulse until well blended and fine, about a minute. Add the melted butter, honey and water and mix until fully combined.
3. Use a spatula to smear the dough on the wax paper. Create a rectangle that is 8 by 11 inches.
4. Bake for 12 minutes, or until browned.
5. Allow to cool completely before cutting into bars. If you're in a hurry (school starts in 30 minutes!) then pick up the wax paper and placeon a cutting board then put it in the freezer. After 5 minutes remove from freezer and cut into bars.

Makes 12 servings

Nutritional Analysis: One serving equals: 154 calories, 14.8g fat, 146mg sodium, 4.5g carbohydrate, 1.6g fiber, and 3g protein.

Raw Apple-Nut Cookies

These cookies are chewy, moist, and great to pack in your lunch or to take on-the-go. Raw cookies are extremely easy to make — there is a huge margin for error, since an extra few hours in the dehydrator won't even make a noticeable difference (as opposed to an extra few minutes in the oven resulting in a tray of charcoal cookies).

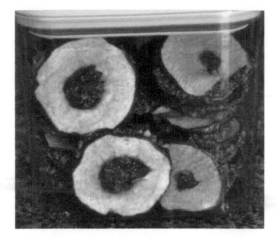

Here's what you need:

- 2 apples, sliced
- 1 cup raw walnuts (soaked 6 hrs, then drained and rinsed)
- 1 cup raw pecans (soaked 6 hrs, then drained and rinsed)
- 2 cups dried figs (soaked 1 hr, then drained and rinsed)
- 1/2 cup dates
- 1 Tablespoon ground cinnamon
- 1 teaspoon salt
- 1 teaspoon nutmeg

1. Cover one dehydrator tray with a non-stick liner.
2. Put the nuts, figs, dates and spices in the food processor, pulse for a few minutes until fully combined. Take a spoonful of dough and press onto a sliced apple, making a round cookie shape. Repeat until all the dough and apple slices have been used.
3. Dehydrate at 115 degrees for 10 hours.

Makes 12 servings

Nutritional Analysis: One serving equals: 254 calories, 14g fat, 134mg sodium, 35.3g carbohydrate, 6.1g fiber, and 3.7g protein.

Real Healthy Apple Pie

This recipe for apple pie is probably different than any you've tried in the past. It's wheat and gluten free, and calls for no sugar. Technically it's a clafoutis, but that sounds a little too pretentious for a pan of baked apples. This pie is lightly sweet and filled with nutritious ingredients. Try it with a dollop of plain or vanilla Greek yogurt.

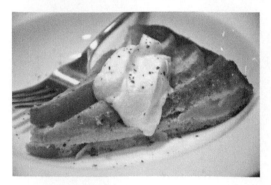

Here's what you need for 12 servings:

- 4-6 medium green apples, cored and sliced
- 4 omega-3, free range eggs
- 2 Tablespoons agave nectar
- 1/2 cup full fat coconut milk, from can
- 2 Tablespoons coconut oil, melted over low heat
- 1 teaspoon vanilla extract
- 1/4 teaspoon almond extract
- 1/3 cup blanched almond flour
- 1/4 teaspoon salt
- 1/2 teaspoon cinnamon plus more for garnish
- Pinch of ground nutmeg

1. Preheat oven to 350 degrees F. Grease a 9-inch pie pan with coconut oil, then dust with blanched almond flour.
2. Arrange the apple spices in concentric circles, fanning out from the center of the pan.
3. In a medium bowl whisk together the eggs, agave nectar, coconut milk, coconut oil, vanilla and almond extracts. In another bowl combine the almond flour, salt, cinnamon and nutmeg.
4. Stir the wet ingredients into the flour mixture until fully combined. Pour over the arranged apples.
5. Bake for 45-55 minutes, until the pie is set and the top is golden. Allow to cool for 30 minutes before slicing.
6. Add a dollop of plain of vanilla Greek yogurt and a sprinkle of cinnamon to each slice.

Makes 12 Servings

Nutritional Analysis: One serving equals: 123 calories, 7g fat, 49mg sodium, 13g carbohydrate, 3g fiber, and 3g protein.

Skillet Apple Pie

Cold winter months make me crave warm sweets, specifically apple pie. I love this Skillet Apple Pie for many reasons. It's super fast, like only 10 minutes. It's sugar and grain free, making it guilt free. And, best of all, it tastes sinfully sweet.

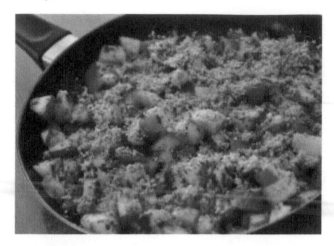

Here's what you need for 3 servings:

- 1 teaspoon coconut oil
- 3 organic apples, try pink lady
- 1 1/2 teaspoons ground cinnamon
- Dash of ground nutmeg
- Dash of sea salt
- 2 Tablespoons golden raisins
- 1/4 cup ground walnuts

1. Melt coconut oil in skillet over medium heat. Wash and chop apples then add to skillet.
2. Cook apples, stirring occasionally, for 5 minutes. Add remaining ingredients, mix and continue to cook until apples are tender.

Makes 3 servings

Nutritional Analysis: One serving equals: 176 calories, 8.2g fat, 78mg sodium, 9g carbohydrate, 3.1g fiber, and 1.7g protein.

Farmer's Market No-Bake Strawberry Pie

After you purchase more Strawberries than you could possibly eat at your local Farmers Market, grab this no-bake strawberry pie recipe and roll up your sleeves. Trust me, the minimal effort needed to crank out this pie is MORE than worth it!

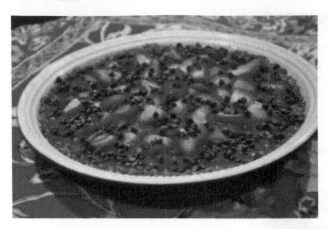

Here's what you need:

- 2 cups pecans
- 1 cup date rolls, or pitted dates
- Dash of salt
- 3 cups strawberries, sliced
- 1 cup strawberries, whole
- 1/3 cup dates, or date pieces, or raisins
- 1 small lemon, juiced
- 1/3 cup Dairy Free Chocolate Chips * optional*

1. Lightly grease pie pan with canola oil. Grind the pecans in a food processor until coarse. Add the date rolls and salt, process until thoroughly combined. Press the mixture into your pie pan.
2. Arrange the sliced berries on the crust. Blend the whole strawberries, dates and lemon juice until smooth. Pour over the sliced strawberries. If you're adding chocolate (and why wouldn't you) then sprinkle over the top of the pie.
3. Refrigerate for about an hour before serving. Note: this pie is best exactly an hour after you make it when the berries are still super fresh, so try to make it right before dinner or right after dinner rather than earlier in the day.

Makes 12 servings

Nutritional Analysis: One serving equals: 299 calories, 16g fat, 31mg sodium, 42.7g carbohydrate, 6.3g fiber, and 3.4g protein.

Real Healthy Berry Crisp with Carmel Cream Topping

Crisps are awesome for sooooo many reasons.

- There's no crust to worry about. Instead you get to crumble the topping with your hands — no way to mess that one up.
- You can use virtually any fruit. There's strawberry and rhubarb crisp in early summer, blueberry crisp in late summer, apple crisp in the fall and then pear crisp. And there are probably other variations that I haven't even tried yet.
- This version of the crisp won't stick to your hips, since I've eliminated the sugar, flour and butter.
- You get to top it with a big spoonful of caramel cream topping...made with Greek yogurt and coconut crystals.

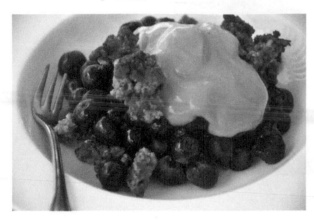

Here's what you need for 10 servings:

- 3 cups fresh berries
- 1 omega-3 egg
- 1 1/2 cups blanched almond meal
- 2 Tablespoons coconut oil, melted
- 2 Tablespoons ground cinnamon
- 1 teaspoon ground nutmeg
- 1 Tablespoon agave nectar OR 1/4 cup coconut crystals
- Carmel Cream topping

1. Preheat oven to 350 degrees F. Lightly grease a pie pan or 8"x8" glass pan with coconut oil.
2. Pour the berries into prepared pan.
3. In a small bowl combine the egg, almond meal, coconut oil, cinnamon, nutmeg and agave nectar (or coconut crystals).
4. Crumble the almond flour mixture by hand evenly over the berries.
5. Bake for 35 minutes.
6. Serve with a dollop of Carmel Cream Topping.

Nutritional Analysis: One serving equals: 164 calories, 11g fat, 13mg sodium, 11g carbohydrate, 3g fiber, and 5g protein.

Carmel Cream Topping

I stumbled upon the perfect recipe for turning plain Greek yogurt into a tasty, dessert-like topping that the kids completely love! And best of all it's low glycemic and filled with vitamins, minerals and protein. Use Caramel Cream Topping on desserts, pancakes, or (my favorite way) by the spoonful.

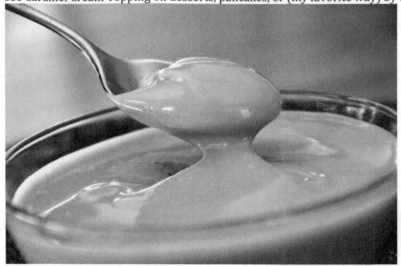

Here's what you need for 36 (1Tablespoon) servings:
- 1 1/2 cups non fat, plain Greek yogurt
- 1/2 cup coconut crystals

1. In a medium bowl, combine 1 cup of the yogurt with the coconut crystals. Mix well, however there will be some balls of coconut crystals.
2. Place in the fridge for 10 minutes.
3. Remove from fridge, mix again. The coconut balls will disappear.
4. Add the remaining 1/2 cup of yogurt to the mixture. Mix well.
5. Serve immediately or chill until you're ready to use.

36 Servings

Nutritional Analysis: One serving equals: 12 calories, 0g fat, 6.2mg sodium, 2g carbohydrate, 0g fiber, and 1g protein.

Guilt-Free Peach Cobbler

After raiding my abundant peach tree, my goal was to create a delicious dessert that wouldn't interfere with my goal to look great at the pool this summer. This guilt-free cobbler is super quick and easy — we are talking about 5 minutes total!

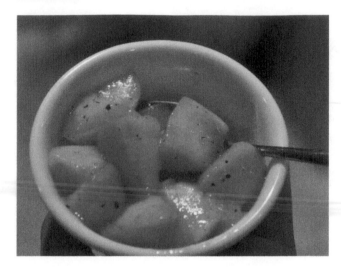

Here's what you need:

- 1 sweet, ripe peach
- coconut cooking spray
- 1 Tablespoon agave nectar
- sprinkle of sea salt
- sprinkle of freshly ground cinnamon

1. Wash, peel and pit the peach. Chop into bite-sized pieces.
2. Pre-heat a skillet over medium-high heat. Spray lightly with coconut cooking spray.
3. Saute the peach pieces for about a minute, then add the agave nectar, salt and cinnamon. Continue to saute for another few minutes until it turns a deep golden color.
4. Serve and enjoy immediately!

Makes 1 serving

Nutritional Analysis: One serving equals: 102 calories, .2g fat, 200mg sodium, 26g carbohydrate, 2.5g fiber, and .9g protein.

Strawberry Fudge Cake

This is one of those recipes that you simply MUST try if you love chocolate. The frosting is especially amazing — don't let the simple, wholesome ingredients fool you.

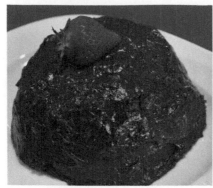 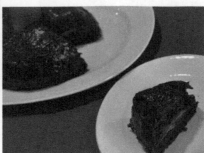

For the cake:

- 3 cups walnuts
- 2/3 cup unsweetened cacao powder
- dash of sea salt
- 1 cup pitted dates
- 2 Tablespoons agave nectar

For the frosting:

- 1/3 cup pitted dates, soaked in hot water for 5 minutes
- 1/4 cup agave nectar
- 1 avocado
- 1/3 cup unsweetened cacao powder

Filling:

- 1/2 cup sliced strawberries

1. Make the cake: Combine the walnuts, cacao powder and salt in food processor or high speed blender. Add the dates and agave nectar and pulse until fully combined. Shape the dough into two round cakes.
2. Make the frosting: Combine the dates and agave nectar in food processor until smooth. Add the flesh from one avocado and the cacao powder. Process until smooth and creamy.
3. Place one of the cakes on cake plate. Frost the top and arrange with sliced strawberries. Place the other cake on top and frost the top and sides. Garnish with strawberry.

Makes 10 servings

Nutritional Analysis: One serving equals: 462 calories, 28.5g fat, 38mg sodium, 60g carbohydrate, 9.6g fiber, and 9.2g protein.

Chocolate Dipped Bananas

Mmmmm, chocolate dipped bananas never tasted as good as they do with this raw vegan chocolate. Freeze bananas ahead of time (my freezer is always stocked with them for the morning green smoothie) and then simply dip in the chocolate, roll on your favorite nut topping and watch as it hardens in about a minute.

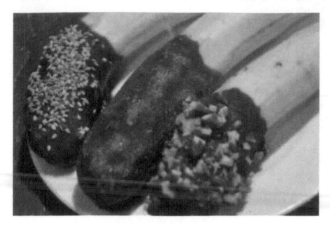

Here's what you need:

For the Raw Vegan Chocolate:

- 1 cup liquid coconut oil (or use cacao butter for a chocolate that won't melt as easily in the sun — liquefy it by placing in a bowl within a bowl of hot water)
- 1/2 cup cacao powder
- 2 Tablespoons agave nectar

1. Place liquefied coconut oil (or cacao butter) in a bowl and mix in the cacao powder and agave.
2. It will last in the fridge for a couple of months, and at room temperature for a few weeks.

For the Frozen Bananas:

- 4 Frozen bananas (you may want to skewer them first)
- Nut toppings

1. Place your nut topping on a plate. Dip the bananas in the chocolate and roll on the toppings.
2. Chocolate will harden within a couple of minutes. If you want to expedite the process, place dipped bananas in the freezer for a minute.

Makes 8 servings (with leftover chocolate)

Nutritional Analysis: One serving equals: 254 calories, 20g fat, 0mg sodium, 17.7g carbohydrate, 2.9g fiber, and 3.6g protein.

Caveman Candy

Here's a super quick recipe for dark chocolate covered figs — aka Caveman Candy. Dried mission figs are packed with natural fiber, vitamins and minerals. It's not often that candy offers you those benefits!

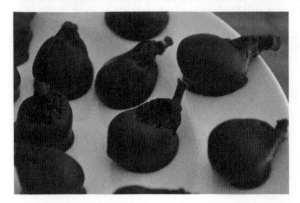

Here's what you need:

- 5 oz dark chocolate — 72% cocoa or higher
- 30 dried mission figs

1. Cover a plate with wax paper and then set aside.
2. Melt the chocolate over very low heat, stirring constantly — or use a double boiler.
3. Grab the figs by their stem and dip into the melted chocolate. Place on the prepared plate.
4. Once all the figs have been dipped, place the plate in the fridge for a least 20 minutes.

Makes 15 servings

Nutritional Analysis: One serving equals: 125 calories, 2.4g fat, 0mg sodium, 27g carbohydrate, 6g fiber, and 3g protein.

Dark Chocolate Almond Bark

Here's a delicious treat that is both good for you and tastes amazing. Dark chocolate is filled with antioxidants and other beneficial properties. Couple that with sliced almonds and a sprinkle of toasted coconut and you've got yourself a splendid treat. Of course enjoy this yumminess in moderation...

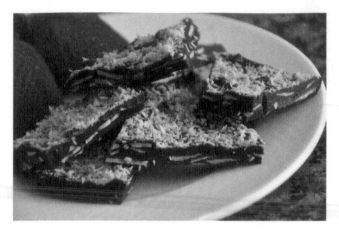

Here's what you need:

- 20 oz dark chocolate, 72% or higher cocoa content
- 1/2 teaspoon almond extract
- 1 cup sliced almonds
- 1/2 cup shredded coconut, lightly toasted

1. Line a tray with wax paper, making sure that it will fit into your freezer.
2. Lightly toast the coconut in a small skillet over low heat. Set aside.
3. Gently melt the chocolate in a double boiler. Mix in the almond extract and sliced almonds. Spread the mixture over the prepared sheet. Evenly sprinkle with coconut.
4. Place in freezer for 30 minutes. Break into pieces.

Makes 20 servings

Nutritional Analysis: One serving equals: 208 calories, 15.6g fat, 12mg sodium, 14.5g carbohydrate, 4.5g fiber, and 3.2g protein.

Chocolate Lover's Pudding

Some days just call for chocolate — you know what I'm talking about! This pudding is quicker to make than instant pudding from a box, and is filled with wholesome nutrients. Kids LOVE this recipe! Treat yourself today.

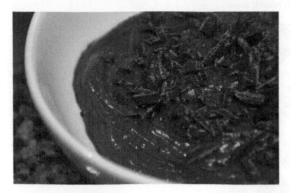

Here's what you need:

- 3 avocados
- 1/4 cup unsweetened cocoa powder
- dash of salt
- 1/2 cup raw honey
- 1 ounce 72% cocoa dark chocolate, finely minced

1. Place avocado flesh, coca powder, salt and raw honey into food processor. Blend until smooth.
2. Serve immediately and top with minced chocolate.

Makes 6 servings

Nutritional Analysis: One serving equals: 256 calories, 15.3g fat, 41mg sodium, 34g carbohydrate, 7.6g fiber, and 2.7g protein.

Real Healthy Strawberry Ice Cream

Here's a strawberry ice cream that you can really get excited about. It's made with 2 simple, wholesome ingredients: organic strawberries and non-fat Greek yogurt.

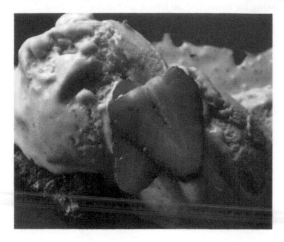

Here's what you need:

- 20 organic strawberries
- 2 cups non fat Greek yogurt

1. Wash and hull the strawberries. Mix in high speed blender until smooth.
2. Add yogurt and blend well.
3. Pour into an ice cream maker and run until yogurt is frozen and creamy.

Makes 2 servings

Nutritional Analysis: One serving equals: 191 calories, 0g fat, 109mg sodium, 24.3g carbohydrate, 5g fiber, and 25.2g protein.

Real Healthy Popsicles

Cure your sweet summer sweet tooth with these wholesome homemade Popsicles!

School is out for the summer months and the kids are constantly asking for Popsicles! So have fun creating your own wholesome Popsicle made with real fruit.

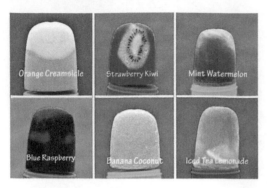

Orange Creamsicle

Here's what you need for 6 servings:

- 2 cups organic, vanilla Greek yogurt
- 1 orange, peeled and seeded
- 1 cup pineapple chunks
- 1 teaspoon agave nectar

1. Fill the bottom 1/3 of each popsicle mold with yogurt. Freeze for 15 minutes.
2. In a high speed blender, combine the orange, pineapple and agave nectar. Blend on high speed for a full minute.
3. Fill the remaining space in each mold with the orange mixture. Freeze until solid.

Makes 6 servings

Nutritional Analysis: One serving equals: 90 calories, 0g fat, 30mg sodium, 15g carbohydrate, 1g fiber, and 8g protein.

_____

Strawberry Kiwi

Here's what you need for 6 servings:

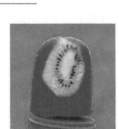

- 2 cups strawberries, hulled
- 2 Tablespoons filtered water
- 2 teaspoons agave nectar (optional)
- 2 kiwis, sliced

1. In a high speed blender, combine the strawberries, water and agave nectar. Allow to run for a full minute on high.
2. Place one slice of kiwi in each popsicle mold, pressed against the side. Fill the molds with the strawberry mixture.
3. Freeze until solid.

Makes 6 servings

Nutritional Analysis: One serving equals: 38 calories, 0g fat, 2mg sodium, 9g carbohydrate, 2g fiber, and 1g protein.

Mint Watermelon

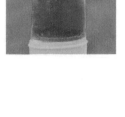

It's easy to make layers by freezing one section at a time. The red and green pattern brings the flavor to life by imitating real slice of watermelon.

Here's what you need for 6 servings:

- 2 cups watermelon pieces
- 3 kiwis, peeled and seeded
- 1 Tablespoon agave nectar
- 30 mint leaves
- 1 Tablespoon filtered water

1. Blend the watermelon in a high speed blender on high for 30 seconds. Fill the bottom 2/3's of each popsicle mold with the watermelon. Freeze for 30 minutes.
2. Combine the kiwi, agave nectar, mint leaves and water in the high speed blender for a full minute or until the tiny pieces of mint have disappeared and the green color is vibrant and uniform.
3. Fill the remaining space in each popsicle mold with the mint mixture. Freeze until solid.

Makes 6 servings

Nutritional Analysis: One serving equals: 42 calories, 0g fat, 3mg sodium, 30g carbohydrate, 2g fiber, and 1g protein.

Blue Raspberry

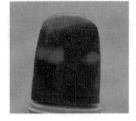

Here's what you need for 6 servings:

- 2 cups blueberries
- 1/4 cup filtered water
- 1 teaspoon agave nectar
- 1 cup raspberries

1. Place the blueberries, water and agave nectar in your high speed blender and blend on high for a full minute or until the little pieces of blueberry skin have disappeared and the purple color is vibrant and uniform.
2. Place 2 whole raspberries in each popsicle mold, then fill with the blueberry mixture. Freeze until solid.

Makes 6 Servings

Nutritional Analysis: One serving equals: 42 calories, 0g fat, 1mg sodium, 10g carbohydrate, 3g fiber, and 1g protein.

Banana Coconut

Here's what you need for 6 servings:

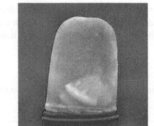

- 2 bananas
- 1 cup coconut milk, full fat from can
- 1/2 cup unsweetened, shredded coconut
- 1 teaspoon agave nectar
- 1 teaspoon ground cinnamon

1. Place the peeled bananas, coconut milk, shredded coconut, agave nectar and cinnamon in your high speed blender. Blend on high for a full minute or until smooth.
2. Fill each popsicle mold. Freeze until solid.

Makes 6 Servings

Nutritional Analysis: One serving equals: 167 calories, 13g fat, 7mg sodium, 13g carbohydrate, 2g fiber, and 2g protein.

Iced Tea Lemonade

Here's what you need for 6 servings:

- 1 cup brewed tea
- 5 dates, pitted
- 1/3 cup lemon juice
- 3 Tablespoons agave nectar
- 1/4 cup water
- decorative lemon slices

1. Brew your tea, then drop the dates in while the tea is still hot. Place the soaking dates in the fridge for 20 minutes.
2. Place the lemon juice, agave nectar, and water in cup and whisk. Set aside.
3. Place the tea and dates in your high speed blender and combine on high for a full minute, or until the tiny date pieces have disappeared.
4. Fill each popsicle mold with a 50-50 combination of tea and lemonade. Add decorative slices of lemon. Freeze until solid.

Makes 6 Servings

Nutritional Analysis: One serving equals: 51 calories, 0g fat, 0mg sodium, 16g carbohydrate, 1g fiber, and .5g protein.

Watermelon Candy

It never ceases to amaze me how much more delicious natural foods are than processed ones. This watermelon candy, which contains only watermelon and lemon juice, has such amazing and satisfying flavor. My kids love these!

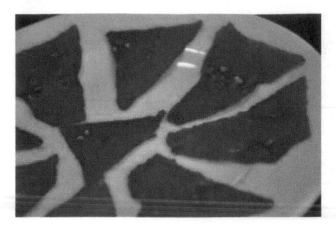

Here's what you need:

- 1 watermelon, sliced into small triangles
- 1 lemons, juiced

1. Slice the watermelon and place in a large bowl. Pour the lemon juice over the watermelon and allow to soak for 10 minutes.
2. Place the watermelon on mesh dehydrator trays. Dehydrate for 12 hours at 110 degrees. Store in an airtight container.

* Tip: Feel free to use extra ripe watermelons for this recipe. Even if the melon is too ripe to enjoy fresh, it will be delicious once dehydrated.

Makes 20 servings

Nutritional Analysis: One serving equals: 60 calories, 0g fat, 2mg sodium, 14.5g carbohydrate, 1g fiber, and 1.2g protein.

Easy Fruit Dessert

Look for the ripest in-season organic fruit and use quality spices for an out-of-this-world taste. The measurements below are vague, this is the kind of recipe that works best when you throw the ingredients together by the handful and sprinkle.

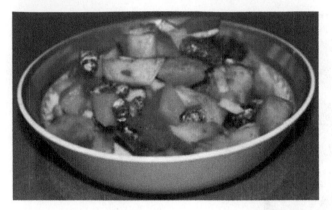

Here's what you need:

- Fresh, organic peaches, nectarines, apples or pears, chopped
- Chopped date pieces
- Jumbo raisins
- Sliced almonds or chopped pecans
- Sprinkle of cinnamon
- A drop of vanilla extract

1. Mix the ingredients together, serve and enjoy immediately.

Tip: Experiment with different combinations of fresh and dried fruits, and, if you're feeling saucy, add a sprinkle of nutmeg

Makes 2 servings

Nutritional Analysis: One serving equals approx. : 250 calories, 5g fat, 2mg sodium, 45g carbohydrate, 6g fiber, and 4g protein.

Real Healthy Poached Pears

If you've never made poached pears, don't be intimidated. The recipe is quite simple, and produces a delicately sweet and delicious treat. Using fresh squeezed oranges instead of sugar, this recipe cuts back on calories and guilt.

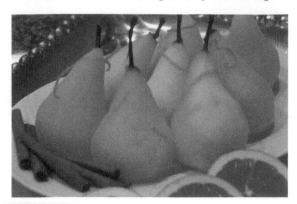

Here's what you need:

- 4 cups fresh squeezed orange juice
- 4 cups water
- 1 (2 inch) piece fresh ginger, peeled
- 6 whole cloves
- 1 cinnamon stick
- zest from an orange
- 6-8 ripe pears
- optional: low fat cottage cheese

1. Place all ingredients, except pears in a large saucepan over low heat.
2. Wash, peel and core the pears. Use a small melon baller to scoop out the core from the bottom of the pear.
3. Place all the pears in the saucepan, making sure that all the pears are fully covered with liquid.
4. Bring the pot to a simmer for 30 minutes. When the pears are soft, but not mushy, remove from liquid.
5. Optional: serve your poached pears over cottage cheese.

Makes 4 servings

Nutritional Analysis: One serving equals approx. (not including cottage cheese) : 172 calories, 0g fat, 4mg sodium, 45g carbohydrate, 7.7g fiber, and 1.3g protein.

CPSIA information can be obtained at www.ICGtesting.com
Printed in the USA
BVOW10s1303091113

335887BV00004B/4/P

9 781888 146011